Soccer Nutrition Handbook

FEED THE CHAMPION IN YOU

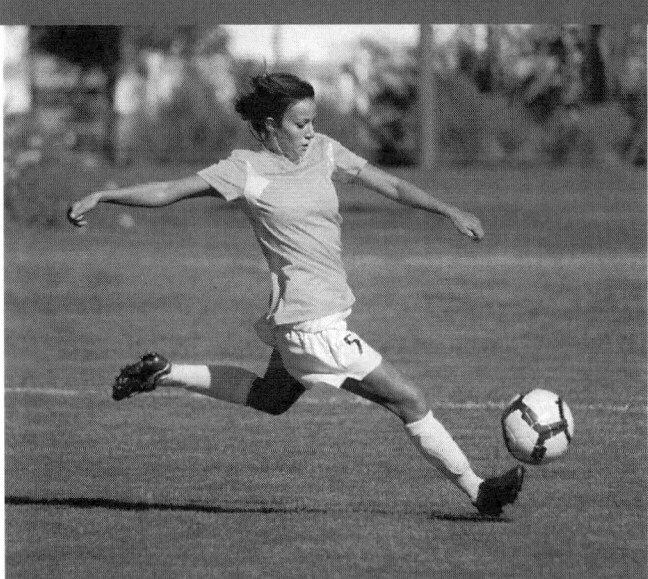

Quick and Easy Personalized Nutrition for Optimum Health and Soccer Performance

Copyright © 2011 by Curt Thompson
All rights reserved.

No part of this publication may be reproduced or transmitted in any form or by any means, electronic or mechanical, including photocopying, and information storage and retrieval systems, without permission in writing from Curt Thompson, Nutrition Coaches, LLC.
ISBN 978-0-615-47178-5
Book cover photography credits:
    www.iStockphoto.com/MIFlippo
    www.IStockphoto.com/Strickke
    www.IStockphoto.com/SJLocke
    www.IStockphoto.com/Majorosl

Disclaimer

The author is not engaged in rendering professional advice or services to the individual reader. The dietary information, programs, resources, ideas, procedures and suggestions contained in this book are not intended as a substitute for consulting with your physician.

You should always consult with your physician before beginning any exercise, dietary or dietary-supplement program. The author is not responsible for your specific health needs, for any allergic or adverse reactions to the dietary programs, suggestions or information contained or referred to in this book, or for any loss or damages arising or allegedly arising from any information or suggestions in this book.

The author has made every effort to provide accurate information and Internet addresses at the time of publication, and does not assume any responsibility for errors or for changes that occur after publication.

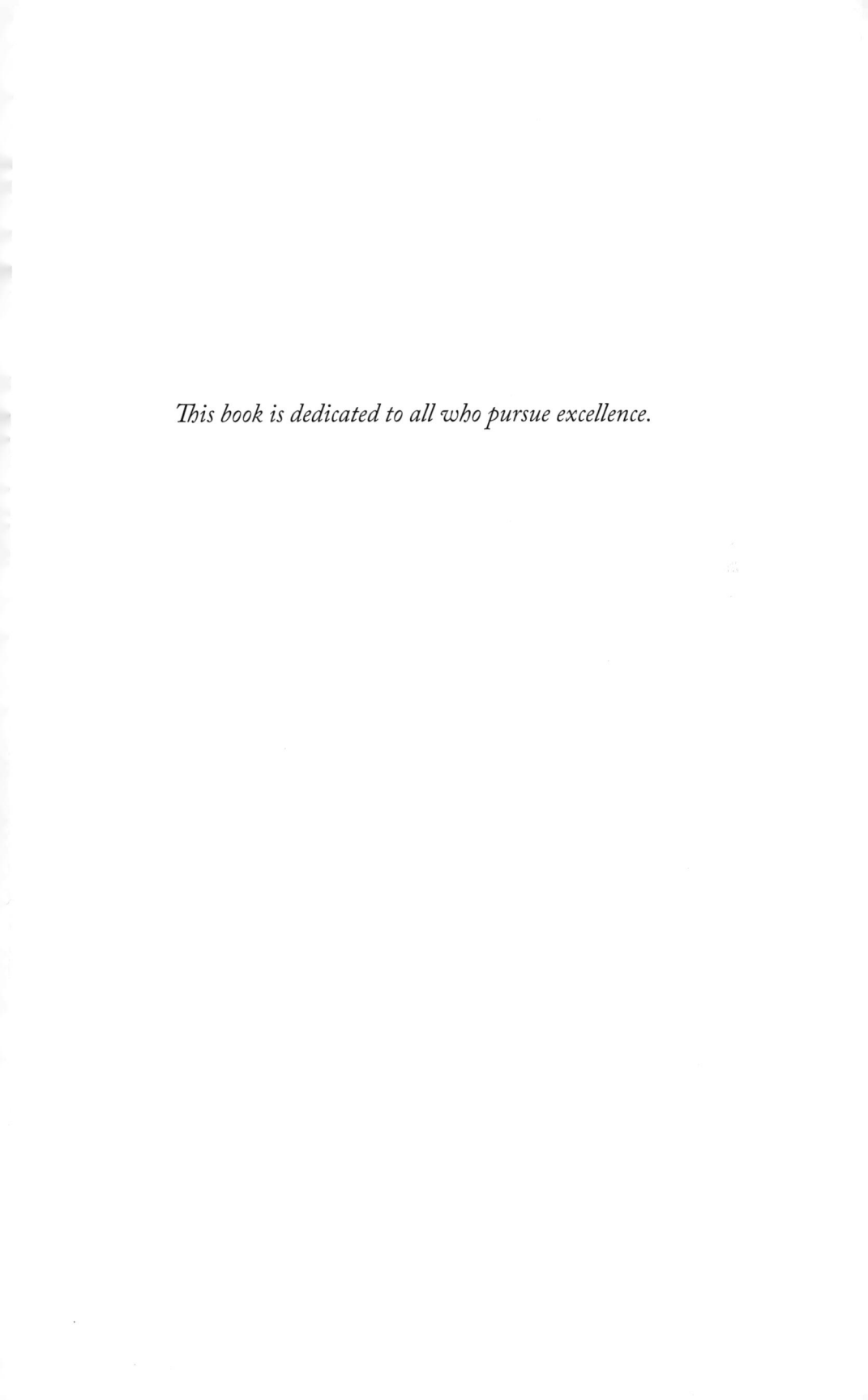

This book is dedicated to all who pursue excellence.

CONTENTS

About the Author ix
Acknowledgments x

HOW TO USE THIS BOOK 1

INTRODUCTION 5
What to Expect 5
Rise Above Your Competition 7
Adjust Your Mindset 8
Commit to Success 8

SECTION I
BECOME YOUR OWN NUTRITION EXPERT 11

Step 1 - Take Control of Your Food 11
Plan Ahead 11
Pack Your Own Lunch and Snacks 12
Eat at Home More Often 12
Learn to Cook 13
Ask Where and How 13
Grow Your Food 14
Step 1 Summary 14

Step 2 - Minimize Sweets 15
The Hidden Danger 15
Recognizing Sugar in Food 18
Artificial Sweeteners 19
Natural Sweeteners 22
Losing Your Sweet Tooth 24
Step 2 Summary 24

Step 3 - Eat Real Food 25
Real Food 25
Industrial Food 27
Food Wisdom 29
Food and Athletic Performance 31
Switching to Whole Foods 32
Preparing Whole Foods 33
The Role of Genetics 33
Step 3 Summary 34

Step 4 - Learn Your Ideal Foods **35**
   The Food Challenge 36
   Day One Food Challenge Instructions 38
   Day One Food Challenge Sample Menu 38
   Day Two Food Challenge Instructions 40
   Day Two Food Challenge Sample Menu 40
   Evaluate Your Food Challenge Results 42
   Using Your Diet Plan 43
   Retesting 43
   Menstrual Cycle (women only) 44
   Step 4 Summary 45

Step 5 - Balance Your Portions **46**
   Diet Plan #1 47
   Diet Plan #2 47
   Diet Plan #1 and #2 Combination 47
   Step 5 Summary 48

Additional Diet Plan Guidelines **49**
   Diet Plan #1 49
   Diet Plan #2 49
   Combination Diet 50
   All Diet Plans 50

From Food to Field: Sensing Your Body's Response **50**

Off and Running **52**

SECTION II
SOCCER SPECIFIC GUIDELINES **53**

Hydration **53**
   How Much to Drink 53
   Choosing the Right Water Bottle 55
   Sports Drinks versus Water 57
   Sport Drink Quality 58

Game Day Nutrition **60**
   Should You Carbohydrate Load? 61

Recovery Food and Drink **63**

Tournament Play **66**
   Before the Tournament 66
   During the Tournament 67
   After the Last Game of the Day 68

Surviving a Fast-Food Situation **69**

Getting the Most From Your Cafeteria **72**

SECTION III

SUPPLEMENTS, SHAKES, BARS AND GOO 77

Supplements 77
Do You Need To Take Nutritional Supplements? 78
Choosing Quality Supplements 78
Which Supplements Should You Take? 81
General Recommendations 82

Shakes, Bars and Goo 88
Protein Powder and Shakes 88
Sport and Energy Bars 90
Goo, Gels, and Shots 90
Energy Drinks 91

SECTION IV

BODY FAT AND PERFORMANCE BLOCKERS 93

Body Fat Management 93
How Much Should I Weigh? 93
How Much Body Fat Do I Need? 94
Body Fat Reduction 95

Food Sensitivity 98
Food Allergy 99
Food Intolerance 101
Checking for a Food Sensitivity 102

Digestive Tract health 104
How Your Digestive Tract Works 105
Digestive tract problems 105

SECTION V

DIETARY FAT DEMYSTIFIED 109

The Role of Fat in the Body 110
What is Fat? 110
Types of Fat 112
Natural, Healthy Fats 113
Unnatural, Industrial Fats 114
Cholesterol 116
The Essential Fats 118
Recommendations for Dietary Fat 123
Summary 127

SECTION VI
MAKE SMART FOOD CHOICES 129

Food Quality 129
Organic 131
Natural or All Natural 131
GMO 131
No Added Hormones or Hormone Free 132
No Antibiotics or Antibiotic Free 132
Free Range *(applies only to poultry animals raised for meat)* 132
Pasture Raised 132
Cage Free 132
Grass Fed (Grass Finished) 132
Grain Fed (Grain Finished) 133

Animal and Seafood Products 133
Cattle, Bison, Sheep 133
Pork 136
Commercial Packaged Meats 138
Chicken and Turkey 138
Eggs 140
Fish and Seafood 142

Produce 145

Dairy 147

Seeds and Tree Nuts 148

Peanuts 149

Grains and Breads 150

Food Preparation, Handling and Storage 152
Meats, Poultry, Fish 153
Fruits and Vegetables 153
Cookware 154
Microwave Cooking 155

SECTION VII
FEED THE CHAMPION IN YOU 159

REFERENCES 163

APPENDIX 171
DIET PLAN 1 – DAILY FOODS 173
DIET PLAN 2 – DAILY FOODS 175
MEAL EVALUATION FORM

About the Author

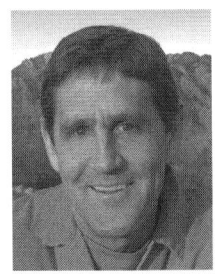

Curt Thompson has provided nutritional counseling to athletes of all ages and sports for over a decade. He holds a Diploma in Comprehensive Nutrition, is a Certified Metabolic Typing Advisor and has a strong background in scientific research. As a motivational speaker, he addresses schools, universities, businesses, community organizations, sports clubs and camps around the country on the critical need for good nutrition.

A nationally licensed soccer coach, Coach Thompson has worked with male and female athletes of all ages and abilities, coaching both youth and adult teams and serving as a soccer camp clinician for 34 years. He has developed numerous unique training methods to build soccer fitness, skill on the ball and game intelligence, and has taught the game of soccer to thousands of players. While doing so he witnessed the damaging effects of poor eating on the health and performance of young athletes. He has now compiled these years of experience, observation and learning into this book on nutrition.

Curt was a walk-on to his college soccer team and graduated four years later as co-captain and Most Valuable Player. Since then, he has captained every team for which he has played and has won eight Colorado state championships and multiple national draw tournaments and league titles. After more than 40 years of playing competitive soccer, he recently retired but still enjoys a kick-around with the youngsters and his wife Beth, who is a soccer coach and a program director at a youth soccer club.

Coach Thompson currently has a private nutrition practice in Boulder, Colorado, and trains aspiring soccer players of all ages through camps, clubs, clinics and private lessons.

ACKNOWLEDGMENTS

I thank the following people for their assistance in the review and preparation of this book:

My wife Beth
My brother Cliff
Dave Oberbillig
Eva Stone
Gina Nicoletti
Dr. Gretchen Sibley
Dr. Jeff Frykholm
John Roberts
Lanie Kohler
Nancy and Ed Widmann
Rachel Hosmer
And the 2010 Centre College Women's Soccer Team

Without their help, patience, contributions and expertise, this book would not exist.

— Curt Thompson—

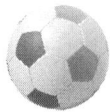

HOW TO USE THIS BOOK

Congratulations! You are about to embark on a journey that will benefit you for the rest of your life. Building health and performance from the inside out is what nutrition is all about, and you now have the best tool for that job.

Your Soccer Nutrition Handbook:

- Is full of practical solutions to common soccer-nutrition problems
- Has concise, easy-to-read paragraphs and quick-to-review bulleted summaries and tables
- Teaches you which foods are "right" for you and which foods to avoid
- Is thoroughly-researched and provides hot links to many useful websites and references should you want to pursue a topic in greater detail

And best part of all, you won't end up buried under a pile of boring technical information.

Here's a quick overview of what you'll find in your *Soccer Nutrition Handbook*:

- **Introduction:** Why nutrition is so important and what to expect.
- **Section I:** Become Your Own Nutrition Expert – a simple, five-step program to personalize your food for optimum performance. This is the core of your Soccer Nutrition Handbook. If you do nothing else, complete this section.

- **Section II:** Soccer Specific Guidelines – addresses topics such as hydration, tournament and game day nutrition, recovery foods, sports drinks and much more.

- **Section III:** Supplements, Shakes, Bars and Goo – practical and cost-effective guidelines on how to choose and use supplements. Also contains a discussion on protein shakes, energy bars and other "energy" products.

- **Section IV:** Body Fat and Performance Blockers – how to manage body fat and identify food sensitivities and other issues that can dramatically affect your health and performance.

- **Section V:** Dietary Fat Demystified – a straight-forward approach to understanding and benefiting from dietary fat.

- **Section VI:** Make Smart Food Choices – how to select, store and prepare healthy foods and avoid common food contaminants.

- **Section VII:** Feed the Champion in You – a book overview and some encouraging words about success.

It is not necessary to read the entire handbook to begin making dietary improvements, but for maximum benefit you must complete the Five Step Program in Section I.

The remainder of the book can be read in the order you choose. Each section is a self-contained discussion about food, drink, soccer performance and health.

It will take time to incorporate the nutrition "skills" you are about to learn into your daily life – the same way it takes time to learn the skills of soccer.

Unless there is a pressing medical need, changing the way you eat should be natural and progressive, like the changing of the seasons.

If you are vegetarian or vegan, you will note that consumption of animal products is discussed in this book.* Don't let that put you off. Instead, do what you do when you read a menu at a restaurant – find the options that work for you – there are many in this handbook.

Eating is a many times per day activity, and there is no better time to start eating well than right now.

So let's get the ball rolling!

---

*Nutrition Coaches, LLC does not encourage or discourage anyone from being vegetarian. Our experience has been that due to genetics, most people are not able to maintain long-term health on a strict plant-based diet, particularly when enduring the physiological demands of playing soccer.

NUTRITION AND YOU

Players

Use the information in this book to build your strength from the inside out. It often helps to get a nutrition buddy to share the experience. If you do nothing else, complete Section I.

You don't need to learn everything in this book to start improving your health and soccer performance, but you do need to be proactive and take control of your food. For example, if your parents buy your food, get them involved in your nutrition program and get yourself involved in your family's food selection and preparation.

Parents

You are the backbone of your family. Therefore, your health and wellness is essential. Set the example for your children, and patiently guide them in the process of learning how to eat well. It will benefit them for the rest of their lives, and will benefit their children as well.

An effective way to do this is to make your children part of family food-selection and preparation experience. Food is and always has been a family-bonding experience. Make it one in your home.

Coaches

Would you let a dehydrated player step onto a soccer field to play in a big game? No! So why do we coaches so often neglect our players' nutrition? Water is just one of many nutrients they need to perform well.

You work hard to train skills and fitness but if your players are malnourished, and many are, much of your effort is wasted. Nutrition is the foundation for your team's performance so make it part of your players' training. It is also a great team-building activity.

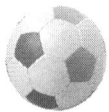

INTRODUCTION

Athletes come in every shape and size – tall, short, slender, heavy, quick, powerful – and from all walks of life and ethnicities. You name it and you will find it on a soccer field.

So why do sport nutrition books treat all athletes exactly the same? Is it really possible that every athlete on Earth, from all the different climates and cultures, can eat exactly the same and perform at his or her best?

Of course not!

You are unique. To power your performance, you need to eat the foods that are "right" for your genetics, not a one-size-fits-all diet plan.

Your *Soccer Nutrition Handbook* will address your individual food needs and show you how to identify the best foods to power your soccer performance and optimize your health.

In short, you are about to become your own nutrition expert.

What to Expect

Consistently eating foods that are "right" for you can yield many benefits:

- Steady and strong daily energy both on and off the field
- Increased endurance and less fatigue after games and practices
- Reduced body fat and improved muscle tone
- Reduced food cravings

- Improved sleep patterns
- Fewer sick days
- An overall sense of well being
- Fewer injuries, faster recovery
- A more positive spirit to endure emotional hardships of tough games and long seasons
- A sharpness of mind to win the "mental moments" that decide games

Just think of how much better a player you will be when you attain all or even some of those benefits.

Your food is the foundation upon which your health and soccer performance is built.

Get that concept in your mind and keep it there. It is a fundamental truth. A second truth is:

Nutrition takes time.

Becoming properly nourished is not a one-day or one-meal event. The human body needs time to process food and nutrients. It needs time to build strength and wellness. Proper nutrition is a long-term, daily activity that, when done correctly, yields fantastic results.

How quickly your body responds depends on several things:
- How well you comply with the guidelines in your *Soccer Nutrition Handbook*
- Your current diet
- Your current state of health
- Your lifestyle habits

Results can often be felt in as little as a few days or a few weeks. In some cases it may take longer. When you consistently eat the foods that are right for you, you will steadily build an unshakeable foundation for your soccer performance.

RISE ABOVE YOUR COMPETITION

It is a fact that many soccer players rarely think about how food affects their performance. To them, food is an afterthought, an unthinking response to hunger.

Here are some common soccer-nutrition questions we field at Nutrition Coaches, LLC:

- What should I eat on game day?
- What should I eat before early morning games or practices?
- Should I drink water or sport drink? And how much?
- What should I eat during tournaments?
- What should I eat after games or hard practices?
- How do I control my body fat?
- What should I eat in the cafeteria?
- Should I take supplements? If so, which ones?

Most of these questions are asked by players who have played soccer for more than 10 years. Clearly, they have not taken the time to learn which foods work best for them. Many never will.

This gives you a huge advantage over your malnourished competition. While they suffer fatigue, higher rates of injury and adopt a "just want practice to end" attitude, the well-fed you will be bright-eyed and ready in both body and spirit to lead the charge against your competition.

Adjust Your Mindset

If you consistently eat poorly, the result will be tired legs, faltering skills, mental mistakes and an increased risk of injury. No amount of training will improve your soccer performance if you are fatigued or injured.

Many athletes reach for quick fixes. It is not uncommon to see soccer players eat junk food day in and day out and then reach for a sugar-laden, caffeine-charged energy drink to get "up" for a game.

> **Fueling Your Game**
>
> Starting a soccer game improperly nourished is self-defeating. Every sprint, shot, header and pass, and every thought and emotion is fueled by what you eat and drink.

This behavior is self-defeating. Despite advertisers' claims, there is no magic pill or miracle in a bottle that can consistently make you play better. Instead, many of those products can cause an energy "crash".

Top soccer players prepare for success by eating well on a daily basis, week after week, season after season. They know that their performance is built on quality nutrition and healthy lifestyle habits, not a miracle in a bottle.

Adjust your mindset right now. To play one of the world's most demanding games, you must eat well on a daily basis.

Commit to Success

To achieve success with your *Soccer Nutrition Handbook* Program, you must give it an honest try. Half-hearted efforts yield half-hearted results. It takes practice to learn a new soccer skill, and your nutrition requires a similar effort.

Pursue the program with a can-do attitude and you will achieve excellent results. Practice your nutrition with the same enthusiasm you practice your soccer skills, and it will quickly become second nature.

In many ways, the program is self-motivating because eating well will make you feel well, and that will make you want to eat well again. Some parts, such as changing your current eating habits, may prove to be challenging, but not overly so.

Nothing about this program should cause anxiety or stress. If it does, you are trying too hard. Step away for a day and put some fun back into the process. Remember, simpler is usually better when it comes to food.

The program can take anywhere from one week to several months to build into your lifestyle. Work at your own pace and remain confident in the outcome.

Don't be shy or worry about what anyone else thinks. And don't for one second think that you need to do what everyone else does to fit in. You don't.

Just as you have your own style on the soccer field, you should have your own style with your food. In fact, your genetic uniqueness makes it essential that you do!

It often helps to do this program with a teammate, friend, parent or sibling. Having a "nutrition buddy" to share the experience can make it that much more enjoyable.

Bottom line: commit to the process and you will learn to properly feed the strong, healthy, fit, happy and clear-thinking player that is in you.

SECTION I

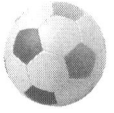

BECOME YOUR OWN NUTRITION EXPERT

The five steps in this section must be completed in order. Do not skip steps. If you only partially complete a step, you will not attain its full benefit, and that may interfere with your ability to successfully complete later steps.

STEP 1 - TAKE CONTROL OF YOUR FOOD

Eating is a many-times-per-day activity that profoundly affects your health and soccer performance. The more other people select and prepare your food, the less you know about what you are putting into your body. When you select and prepare your food, you control what goes into your body.

Plan Ahead

Most people end up at fast food restaurants because they haven't taken the time to think ahead. This puts them in a position of having to eat whatever is available when they get hungry, and often that is not a quality meal.

With just a little planning, you can have healthy food available to you at home, work, school or when traveling. An effective way to do this is to take three minutes each evening and answer the following questions:

- What time do I need to wake up to have enough time to eat breakfast?
- What am I going to eat for breakfast?

- What snacks will I need to bring with me?
- When in my schedule can I eat those snacks?
- What food and drink do I need before and after my soccer practice or game?

Answer these questions in advance and you will be "food prepared" each day.

Pack Your Own Lunch and Snacks

Being hungry near a vending machine usually results in unhealthy eating. However, if you have a healthy snack with you, that is not a problem. Let the vending machine go hungry.

Lunch is often away from home, either at work or school. The best lunch is the one you prepare at home and bring with you. Fail to prepare a lunch and chances are you will be eating lower-quality food prepared by someone else.

Eat at Home More Often

Buying and preparing your own food is an easy and effective way to take control of your food. It is not always possible, but the more you do it the better.

Restaurant and fast-food workers are motivated far more by monetary profit than by your wellness. It is not uncommon to hear a restaurant worker say, "If you knew what went on in the kitchen, you wouldn't eat at this restaurant."

Here are some common reasons that cause restaurants to fail safety and health inspections:

- Failure to restrict ill employees from handling food
- Failure of employees to wash their hands – for example, after using restroom
- Employees touching ready-to-eat foods with their bare hands

- Failure to cook raw meats to a safe temperature
- Cross contamination between raw (uncooked) and ready-to-eat foods
- Failure to sanitize equipment and utensils
- Presence of rodents and pests

Clearly, from the perspective of health alone, you are the best person to prepare your food.

This does not mean you never go out to eat again. Restaurant dining is wonderful for special occasions and socializing. In some cases, such as business meetings or travel, it is essential.

However, if you eat away from home more than at home, then someone else is more in control of your food than are you.

Another benefit is the money you can save by preparing your food. Spending just $20 per week in a restaurant adds up to more than a $1,000 dollars per year. A better use of that money might be to buy higher quality food to eat at home.

Learn to Cook

If you don't already know how to cook, take some time to learn. Everyone should know how to prepare food. It has been an essential survival skill since man has been walking upright.

Keep your cooking simple. Healthy eating does not require gourmet preparation.

In Section VI of your *Soccer Nutrition Handbook*, you will find some basic food preparation guidelines that will allow you to obtain maximum nutrient content from your food.

Ask Where and How

Ask those handling your food where it comes from and how it is prepared. If you don't ask, you won't know. Some of the answers may surprise you.

Grow Your Food

It's not always practical, but growing some of your own food is a very healthy and rewarding activity.

Step 1 Summary

- Take control of your food – know your food's source, quality and cleanliness.
- As much as possible control the handling and preparation of your food from source to mouth.
- Plan ahead, learn to cook and pack you own lunch and snacks.
- Eat at home more often than out.
- If possible, grow some of your food.

STEP 2 - MINIMIZE SWEETS

Of all the foods in the modern diet, refined sugar is one of the least beneficial and most pervasive. It takes many forms and, when consumed in excess, disrupts body chemistry and devastates the immune system.

Dietary sugar has also been implicated in:[1]

- Allergies
- Anxiety issues
- Arthritis
- Blood sugar imbalances
- Chronic inflammation
- Diabetes
- Fatigue
- Heart disease
- Mood problems
- Obesity
- Reduced tissue elasticity
- Weakened bones
- And many other disorders

These conditions do not build healthy, fit and clear-thinking soccer players.

Nutrition Coaches, LLC has yet to find a client who hasn't dramatically benefitted, both on and off the field, from reducing sugar intake.

The Hidden Danger

Dietary sugar can be "natural," like that found in fruit, or "added," like that found in non-diet soda and cake frosting.

When consumed in its natural form, such as in whole fruit, sugar can be a healthy source of energy. However, if you regularly consume large amounts of unhealthy, added sugars, your soccer performance can be significantly diminished.

Unfortunately, a lot of sugar is "hidden" in everyday food and drink.

For example:

- In one 3-teaspoon serving of ketchup there is 1 teaspoon of sugar.
- In one can of non-diet soda there can be as many as 14 teaspoons of sugar.
- One cup of breakfast cereal can contain 6 teaspoons of sugar.

Total Sugar Content of Some Common Food and Drink*

Food or Drink	Amount	Sugar Content (teaspoons)
Bagel	1 bagel	1-2
Bread	1 slice	1-2
Candy bar	1 bar	2-8
Cereal, breakfast	1 cup	2-6
Cookie	2 cookies	2-6
Doughnut	1 doughnut	2-6
Drinks		
Energy Drink (non-diet)	8 fl oz	5-8
Fruit juice	8 fl oz	4-12
Soda (non-diet)	12 fl oz (1 can)	8-14
Sport Drink	8 fl oz	5-6
Granola / cereal / sport bars	1 bar	2-5
Ice cream	½ cup	3-8
Milk	8 fl oz	3
Milkshake, Fast Food	12 fl oz	9-24
Muffin or cupcake	1 cake	2-6
Pancakes with syrup	1 serving	6-12
Oatmeal, instant	1 pkg	2-4
Pie	1/8 pie	5-12
Yogurt	6 oz	2-10

*Data summarized from USDA Database for the Added Sugars Content of Selected Foods, Release 1, February 2006, and Appleton, N. Lick the Sugar Habit Sugar Counter. Penguin Putnam, 2001.

Have a bowl of sweetened cereal for breakfast and wash down your lunchtime French Fries and ketchup with a can of soda and you have already eaten nearly 20 teaspoons of sugar.

Twenty teaspoons is an immense amount of sugar. The American Heart Association recommends that adult men and women limit consumption of added sugar to nine and six teaspoons per day, respectively.[2]

Multiple surveys performed by Nutrition Coaches, LLC on young soccer players show they commonly consume 50 to 70 teaspoons of sugar per day, most of it from sweet beverages such as sodas, sweet teas, flavored milk, coffees, juices and sport drinks.

That works out to between 160 and 225 pounds of sugar per year!

For many young players, that is twice their body weight!

Consuming that much sugar on a daily basis is a disaster when it comes to health and soccer performance.

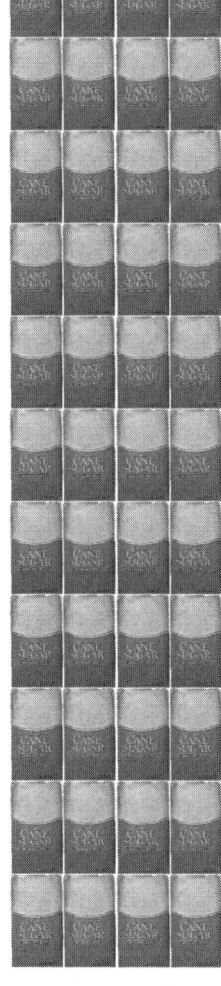
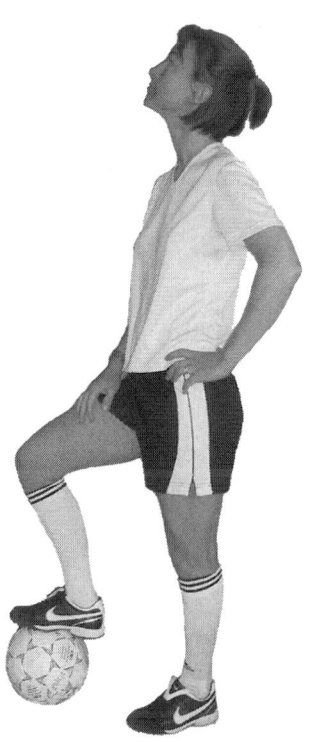

A 110-pound player next to 44 five-pound bags (220 pounds) of sugar.

Recognizing Sugar in Food

Added sugar can take many forms, such as:

- High fructose corn syrup (HFCS)
- Concentrated fruit juice and syrups
- Sucrose (table sugar)
- Fructose (fruit sugar)
- Lactose (milk sugar)
- Maltose (grain sugar)
- Dextrose
- Brown sugar
- Maple sugar and syrup
- Beet juice
- Molasses
- Honey

You will need to read food labels to identify how much sugar a food contains. Sugar is listed under "Carbohydrates." The quantity is in grams per serving.

There are approximately four grams of sugar per teaspoon.

To calculate how many teaspoons of sugar there are in one serving of a food, simply divide the number of grams of sugar by four.

However, to determine how much sugar is in the entire package of food you must multiply that result by the number of servings per package.

A label from a 20-ounce bottle of sport drink illustrates this point.

Ingredients

Water, Sucrose, High Fructose Corn Syrup, Salt, Citric Acid, Natural Flavors, Salt, Sodium Citrate, Monopotassium Phosphate, Ester Gum, Red 40, Carmel Color

Nutrition Facts

Serving Size 8 fl oz. (240 ml)
Servings Per Container 2.5

Amount Per Serving
Calories 50

	% Daily Value
Total Fat 0 g	0%
Sodium 110 mg	5%
Potassium 30 mg	1%
Total Carbohydrate 14g	5%
Sugars 14g	
Protein 0 g	

In this sport drink there are 14 grams of sugar per serving. However, there are 2.5 servings per bottle. If you drink the entire bottle, as most people do, you will consume nearly nine teaspoons of sugar – from both sucrose and high fructose corn syrup.

Virtually all of the sugar in this sport drink is added. Unfortunately, you can't always identify how much added sugar is in a food just by looking at the label. For example, chocolate milk will often contain natural sugar from the milk and added sugar from the chocolate flavoring.

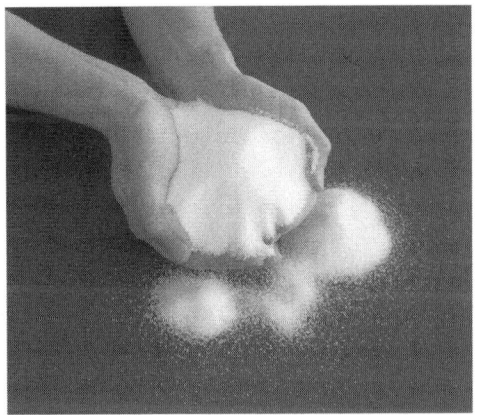

The best approach when choosing foods is to select those that are low in total sugar and have no additional forms of sugar in the ingredient list. More information about the added sugar content of common foods can be found with an online search for "USDA Database for the Added Sugar Content of Selected Foods."

The equivalent amount of sugar in a large vanilla milkshake from a popular fast-food restaurant.

(www.ars.usda.gov/services/docs.htm?docid=12107)

Artificial Sweeteners

By now you may be thinking about switching to artificial sweeteners instead of sugar. Don't!

A simple Internet search reveals the controversy surrounding the possible negative health effects of artificial sweetener use. Manufacturers claim their products are completely safe and back it up with scientific studies. Opponents claim the exact opposite and also provide scientific studies.

Here are some of the top complaints from users of artificial sweeteners:

- Anxiety attacks
- Breathing difficulty
- Depression
- Dizziness
- Fatigue
- Headache/migraine
- Hearing loss
- Heart palpitation
- Insomnia
- Irritability
- Joint pain
- Memory loss
- Muscle spasms
- Nausea
- Numbness
- Rashes
- Seizures
- Slurred speech
- Vision problems
- Weight gain

One well-noted researcher has linked aspartame, the sweetener found in many diet drinks and sugar-free products, to brain and neurological damage and an increase in the risk of brain tumors in children.[3]

And when it comes to weight loss, the authors of a Purdue University study concluded that consuming a food sweetened with an artificial sweetener can actually have an opposite effect and lead to a greater gain in body fat than would a food sweetened with sugar.[4]

In other words, you are better off eating a sugar-sweetened food than an artificially sweetened "diet" food if you want to lose body fat!

Another problem with artificial sweeteners is that their intense sweetness makes naturally-sweet, healthy foods, such as fruit, less appealing – a situation that can lead to an overall reduction of diet quality.

The controversy over artificial sweeteners rages on. When so much controversy exists about a product, the safest approach is to simply avoid it until it is proven to cause no harm over a long period of time.

Here is a list of common artificial sweeteners and some of their brand names to help you identify them on food ingredient labels:

- Acesulfame K or Ace K (Sweet One, Sweet-n-Safe, Sunette)
- Aspartame (Nutrasweet, Equal, AminoSweet, NatraTaste Blue)
- Neotame
- Saccharin (Sweet 'n Low, Sugar Twin)
- Sucralose (Splenda)
- Sugar alcohols (Sorbitol, Xylitol, Mannitol, Maltitol)

These artificial sweeteners can commonly be found in:

- Baked goods
- Candy (sugar free)
- Chewing gum (most)
- Diet sodas
- Energy bars
- Flavored waters
- Frozen foods
- Ice cream and frozen treats
- Jams and jellies (low / sugar free)
- Juices (low or zero calorie)
- Low calorie yogurt
- Sport drinks

If you are uncertain if a product contains an artificial sweetener, here is a simple rule:

If a food or drink tastes sweet and has little or no sugar listed on the label, it probably has an artificial sweetener in it.

It is the opinion of Nutrition Coaches, LLC that unless there is a compelling medical reason for you to consume artificial sweeteners, they are best avoided.

Natural Sweeteners

If you occasionally use a sweetener for baking or flavoring food and drink, choose a more natural form rather than highly-processed white sugar. Even though these products are more natural, they should still be used in moderation.

Raw Sugar

Unrefined raw sugar contains traces of nutrients that are stripped from white sugar and brown sugar during processing. These minerals include phosphorus, calcium, iron, magnesium, and potassium.

> **Baking Tip**
>
> When baking, the amount of sugar in a recipe can often be cut in half with little effect on taste. Give it a try!

In addition, unrefined sugar is free of the potentially harmful chemicals often used in processing white sugar, such as sulphur dioxide, phosphoric acid, etc.

Raw sugar is brown in color but is not the same as brown sugar. Brown sugar is a combination of processed sugar and molasses.

Raw sugar can be substituted for white sugar in many baking recipes but its large crystals may need to be dissolved first.

Honey

In its raw, unfiltered, unheated form, honey is a healthy sweetener that has many beneficial properties. Since ancient times, some of its more traditional uses have been:

- To treat upset stomach conditions
- As a topical burn and skin-wound treatment
- To reduce cough due to illness

- To improve immune function
- To reduce allergy and asthma symptoms

However, due to the risk of infant botulism, honey should not be given to children younger than 12 months of age. Parents of infants should also be wary of baked goods and cereals that are honey-flavored.

Honey is nearly twice as sweet as sugar, so it should be used sparingly.

Pure Maple Syrup

Pure maple sugar is three times sweeter than white sugar and has fewer calories. It also contains manganese, zinc and antioxidants that support immune system function.

Maple syrup can add a unique flavor to many foods and drink such as tea, oatmeal, baked goods and even cooked sweet potatoes.

Due to its inherent sweetness, maple sugar is also best used sparingly.

Stevia

This South American herb has been used as a natural sweetener by traditional cultures for hundreds of years. No significant health effects have been noted when it is used in moderation.

Stevia is sold as a supplement in both liquid and powder form and is about 30 times sweeter than sugar. Diabetics often use it because it has minimal effects on blood sugar levels.

Stevia has a wide variation in its taste between brands, and you may need to try several brands before you find one you like. When used in moderation, Stevia can be an acceptable natural alternative to sugar.

Losing Your Sweet Tooth

Sugar is powerfully addictive and if you are "hooked" on sugar you may go through a withdrawal of sorts when you stop consuming it.[5]

This process of losing your sweet tooth may be challenging, but once you get the sweet food and drink out of your diet for a few weeks, your taste buds will reset themselves and your cravings for sweets will diminish.

Then, those same intensely sweet foods that you used to crave will taste far too sweet, and less-sweet natural foods, such as whole fruit, will again taste as they were meant to taste.

Step 2 Summary

- Reduce added sugars to less than 6 teaspoons per day for females; 9 teaspoons for males (remember: 4 grams of sugar per teaspoon).
- Read labels to determine sugar content of food.
- Avoid artificial sweeteners unless required for medical reasons.
- Use raw honey, pure maple syrup and Stevia as sugar alternatives (honey should not be given to babies under one year of age).

Step 3 - Eat Real Food

Real Food

Real foods or whole foods are those that are or were recently alive and growing, as close as possible to their natural form, and minimally processed. An example of a real food is a strawberry. Strawberry jam is a highly processed food made from strawberries.

A Plate of Real Food

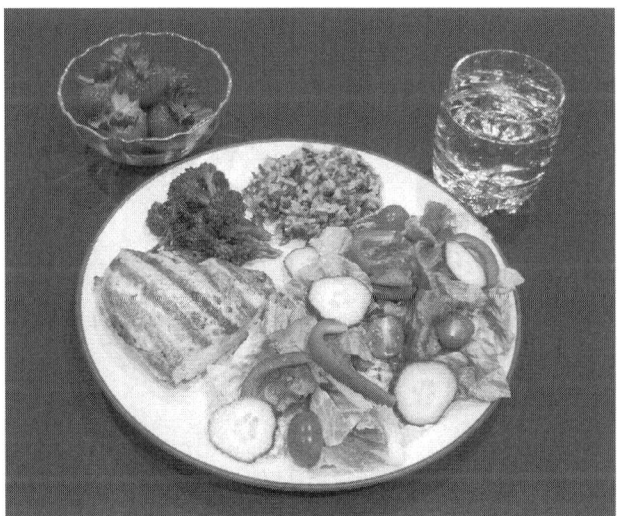

Ingredients
(minus condiments)
Chicken breast
Broccoli
Wild rice
Lettuce
Cucumber
Red pepper
Tomato
Strawberries
Blueberries
Filtered water
Ten healthy ingredients

Here are some other common examples of real foods:

- Eggs (whole)
- Fish, Chicken and Turkey
- Beef, Bison and Pork
- Vegetables
- Fruits
- Nuts and Seeds
- Legumes (beans)
- Whole grains:
  - Wheat
  - Wild rice
  - Oats
  - Quinoa

A Plate of Industrial Food

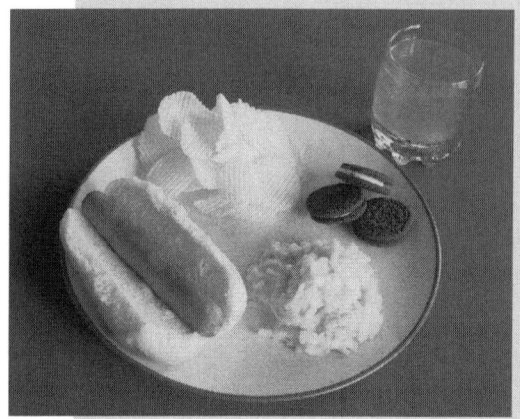

Ingredients (minus condiments)

HOTDOG: beef, water, salt, sorbitol, potassium lactate, sodium diacetate, flavorings, sodium phosphates, sodium erythrobate, sodium nitrate

BUN: enriched flour, water, high fructose corn syrup, soybean oil, yeast, salt, sodium stearoyl lactylate, mono-& diglycerides, ammonium sulfate, calcium propionate, wheat gluten, calcium sulfate, mono calcium phosphate, calcium carbonate, ascorbic acid, azodicarbonamide, enzymes, soy lecithin

MACARONI & CHEESE: wheat flour, clyceryl monostearate, niacin, ferrous sulfate, thiamin mononitrate, riboflavin, folic acid, whey, corn syrup solids, palm oil, milk, milk fat, milk protein concentrate, salt, sodium tripolyphosphate, medium chain triglycerides, maltodextrin, dried buttermilk, sodium phosphate, citric acid, guar gum, high acid whey, cream, lactic acid, calcium phosphate, cheese culture, skim milk, modified food starch, yellow 5, natural flavor, yellow 6, enzymes, annatto, artificial flavor, salt, maltodextrin, potassium chloride, acetylated monoglycerides, medium chain triglycedrides, citric acid, apocarotenal

POTATO CHIPS: potatoes, sunflower oil and/or corn oil, salt

COOKIES: sugar, wheat flour, niacin, reduced iron, thiamine mononitrate, riboflavin, folic acid, high oleic canola oil and or palm oil and/or canola oil, and/or soybean oil, cocoa, high fructose corn syrup, corn starch, baking soda and/or calcium phosphate, salt, soy lecithin, artificial flavor, chocolate

JUICE: water, apple and grape juice concentrate, calcium lactate, pineapple, orange and cherry juice concentrate, natural flavor, ascorbic acid

How many of these 100-plus ingredients are "healthy"?

Industrial Food

Industrialized food processing began in earnest near the end of World War II and has been escalating ever since.

The family farm has been replaced by huge agricultural operations. Livestock is now processed in giant industrial feedlots, and chickens and turkeys are grown by the millions in huge warehouses. Fish that used to swim freely in the ocean are now raised in massive, floating fish farms.

The low cost and convenience of industrial foods is impressive. They are produced in huge quantities at blinding speeds and delivered in pre-cooked or microwave-ready, eat-on-the-go serving sizes and eye-catching packaging.

The cheaper and faster a food is made and sold, the greater the profit. This has pushed the preservation of the nutrient quality of food to a low priority and consequently, industrial foods are often loaded with taste-bud pleasing calories but are short on health-building nutrients.

Here are some common examples of processed (industrial) foods:

- Doughnuts and French fries
- Soft drinks and many flavored waters
- Chips, cookies, crackers and candy
- Sugar, high fructose corn syrup
- Non-whole grain breads
- White rice and most pastas
- Most breakfast cereals
- Many commercial fruit and vegetable juices
- Most sport and energy drinks
- Most sport and energy bars
- Most commercial baked goods
- Most commercial soups
- Processed meats (hot dogs, sausage, most cold cuts, etc.)

Here is a nutrition label and ingredient list from a commercially-produced jar of strawberry jam.

Ingredients

Strawberries, High Fructose Corn Syrup, Corn Syrup, Sugar, Fruit Pectin, Citric Acid

Nutrition Facts

Serving Size 1 tbsp (20g)

Amount Per Serving

Calories 50

	% Daily Value*
Total Fat 0 g	0%
Total Carbohydrate 13g	4%
Sugars 13g	
Protein 0 g	

Vitamin A	0%	Calcium	0%
Vitamin C	0%	Iron	0%

As you can see, the primary ingredient is strawberries, followed by three sweeteners, a thickener (pectin) and a preservative (citric acid).

A strawberry in its whole, just-picked form is highly nutritious, containing vitamins A, C and B6, fiber, potassium, folate and various antioxidants, enzymes and many trace amino acids.

The label on this particular jar of strawberry jam was colorfully decorated with eye-catching pictures of bright red, whole strawberries. At first glance, it is easy to conclude that this product contains the wholesome nutrition of whole strawberries.

But a critical look at the nutrition label reveals a completely different story.

There are negligible amounts of vitamin A, C and calcium and iron in the finished jam, and according to a representative of the company that made the jam, there are no other measureable nutrients.

A look at the sugar content reveals that a one tablespoon serving contains the equivalent of one tablespoon of sugar. In other words, this jam is nothing more than a taste-pleasing lump of strawberry-flavored sugar.

Fresh, nutrient-rich strawberries go into the factory and sugar-laden, nutrient-free jam comes out. Somewhere in the middle, the powerful health-promoting nutrients of the whole strawberry are completely eliminated.

Sadly, most of the thousands of industrial food products that line supermarket shelves are nutrient depleted.

Why does that matter?

Turning food into body energy requires many different nutrients working in concert. If your food doesn't provide them, your body will draw from its own nutrient stores to get the job done.

For example, if your body needs calcium and you are not getting enough dietary calcium, it will pull what it needs from your calcium reserves, otherwise known as your bones.

Pull calcium from your bones too often for too long and they will become brittle and weak. And with nutrient depletion being such a gradual process, chances are you won't feel a thing until it's too late.

This is just one possible consequence of regularly eating foods that are nutrient imbalanced. Add in the nutritional demands of hard soccer training and a small imbalance becomes a big problem.

You need more than just energy from your food.

You also need nutrients.

Food Wisdom

Thousands of years ago, your ancestors lived and thrived on the foods they found in Nature.

Hunting, gathering and preparing food was the prime daily activity of men, women and children alike, with great care being taken to obtain foods of the highest nutrient quality.

Food knowledge was passed from generation to generation because that knowledge was the key to survival. Family life often revolved around food, and food played a powerful role in the development of cultures.

Now, industrial foods are so prolific that food has become a grab-and-go thing, with many families not even coming together for one meal a day. Gone are the days of food being a top priority in family life.

Fast-food restaurants are on nearly every major street corner and industrial foods dominate supermarket shelves. Many people now eat away from home far more than at home.

> **Children and Food**
>
> The more children are involved in gathering and preparing food, the smarter they will be about food as adults and parents.
>
> A good way to get them involved is have children over the age of 12 plan and prepare one healthy family meal each week.

Many parents do not know the basics of how to prepare healthy food, choosing instead to buy microwavable dinners for their children.

The extent of cooking knowledge in teenage and college-age soccer players is often limited to boiling water for noodles, dropping frozen waffles in a toaster or microwaving chicken nugget things.

So little thought is given to food and nutritional value that many children are unable to recognize common fruits and vegetables or tell you where an egg comes from. Even less thought is given to how food affects health and athletic performance.

This dumbing-down of nutritional wisdom has had its consequences. The high rates of obesity, diabetes, and heart disease plaguing our world are primarily the result of industrial foods replacing whole-food diets.[6]

But as grim as our modern food world appears, it is important to keep in mind that even though our supermarkets are filled with industrial foods, they are also full of whole foods such as fruits, vegetables, eggs, meat and fish. And thanks to modern transportation, whole foods are available to you nearly every day of the year.

So the next time you go hunting and gathering food at your local supermarket, here are two nuggets of food wisdom to keep mind:

- You don't have to change the world to eat well – you just have to make better personal food choices.
- If your ancient ancestors wouldn't recognize it as food, you probably shouldn't eat it.

Food and Athletic Performance

Your soccer performance and health are dependent on the energy you obtain from food and drink. Energy in food takes the form of protein, fat and carbohydrate.

Converting food energy into a form that your body can use is a complex process requiring a host of supporting nutrients such as vitamins, minerals, antioxidants, enzymes and phytochemicals.

The right combination of food energy and nutrients turns each of your trillions of cells into a body-energizing factory.

The wrong combination can leave you feeling physically, mentally and emotionally drained.

Whole foods naturally provide the right balance of energy and nutrients for top athletic performance. They are what your body is genetically designed to eat.

> **Phytochemicals**
>
> Phytochemicals, sometimes called phytonutrients, are plant-based chemicals that impart tastes, aromas, colors and other characteristics to food.
>
> They act as antioxidants, hormone regulators and help defend against cancer and heart disease.
>
> Carotenoids and flavanoids are two common phytochemicals.

Industrial foods, apart from being nutrient poor, often contain added chemicals such as artificial flavors, colors and preservatives, which can cause a host of health and performance problems.

Simply put, your body is not designed to thrive on industrial foods. It can handle them in limited quantities but if they are your primary food source, your performance on a soccer field will be far below what it could be.

Switching to Whole Foods

Switching to whole foods may take some adjustment. One approach is to completely clear your home or place of residence of industrial foods and start fresh with whole foods.

If this seems a little extreme – and for most people it is – slowly phase out the majority of industrial foods and ease into more whole foods over a month or two. How you make the transition is your choice.

> **The goal is to make your home or place of residence a healthy refuge amid the junk-food squalor of the modern food world.**

It is difficult to eat well at every meal. A reasonable goal is to make 18 out of 21 meals each week "healthy".

> **The 18-21 Rule**
> Make 18 out of 21 meals each week "healthy".

Holidays, special events and birthdays are often times when less-healthy food is served. Make those your non-healthy meals and get back on track the next meal or day.

If you are on a cafeteria meal plan or one or more of your daily meals are from a dining hall or cafeteria, then it becomes a matter of choosing the best foods available. See Getting the Most from Your Cafeteria in Section II for how to make good cafeteria-food choices.

Preparing Whole Foods

Whole foods can take a little more time to prepare than industrial foods, however, the long-term gains in health and performance will far exceed the effort put into that preparation (see Food Selection and Preparation Guidelines in Section VI).

Many fruits and vegetables are best consumed raw. In addition to vitamins and minerals, raw foods contain enzymes that assist in the digestion and absorption of the food nutrients and thousands of phytochemicals, which support all body functions and work to suppress disease such as cancer.[7,8,9]

In addition to vitamins B and C, many of these "other" nutrients are degraded or destroyed by cooking.

To ensure you are getting a sufficient quantity and variety of nutrients in your diet, you should consume one third or more of your food in raw form. A common approach is to eat more raw foods in the summer and less in the winter as raw foods tend to cool the body and cooked foods warm the body.

Whole fruits and salads are a great way to get a raw food into your diet, as are raw nuts and seeds such as almonds, pecans, sunflower seeds, etc.

The Role of Genetics

For thousands of generations, humans have by necessity adapted to live in various climates with vastly different sources of whole food.

Eskimos eat a high fat and protein diet. South Pacific Islanders eat coconuts, fruit and reef fish.

Those that failed to adapt to their environment did not survive.

Your ancestors were the survivors. The genetic program they passed along to you means you are likely to thrive on what they ate.

Maybe in a few thousand years humans will adapt to thrive on industrial foods but until then, your best foods are the whole foods your ancestors ate. And there is no changing that fact.

You can't ask your ancestors what they ate, but there is an easy way to learn which foods work best for you. This is what you will accomplish next in Step 4.

Step 3 Summary

- You are genetically designed to eat and thrive on real (whole) foods.
- Real foods naturally combine the energy and nutrients needed for health and top athletic performance.
- Minimize consumption of industrial foods. As a general rule, the more a food is processed, the less healthy it is for you.
- Follow the 18-21 Rule – make 18 out of 21 meals each week healthy.
- Consume one third or more of your food in raw form (fruit, vegetables, nuts, seeds).

Step 4 - Learn Your Ideal Foods

Once real foods comprise the majority of your diet, you will have taken a huge step toward giving your body what it needs to perform at its best. However, to fully maximize your health and soccer performance, you need to identify which whole foods work best for you.

Some athletes perform better on a higher protein and fat diet while others do better on a higher carbohydrate diet. Some perform well on a balanced mix of the two. Furthermore, the type of protein, such as red or white meat, can also play a very powerful role.

The genetic difference between people determines how each individual processes and uses food to generate body energy.[10,11,12,13] Consequently, what powers one person's top performance may or may not power yours.

For example, if you eat lunch and an hour or two later you can't keep your eyes open and feel foggy-headed or moody for no particular reason; your lunch did not provide your cells with what they needed to properly energize you.

However, if you eat lunch and for the next four or five hours you feel energetic, clear thinking and of good spirit, your lunch provided a lasting, effective source of energy for your trillions of cells.

Eat three meals like that and the whole day becomes a health-building, energy-packed experience.

> **Given the right nutrition, your cells are able to do exactly what they are designed to do – energize your body and mind to be alert, spirited and strong. This is how your body signals to you that you ate the "right" foods.**

Unfortunately, this body-feedback signal is often ignored. For most people, when a meal leaves them feeling tired and down, they simply eat more of the exact same food that made them feel tired and down in the first place. Many also reach for caffeine as a "pick-me-up", which may explain the appearance of coffee shops on nearly every street corner.

As a result, each wrong-food day knocks a little chip off the foundation that supports health and performance.

Soccer players are no different. Most do not understand the powerful connection between food and performance and end up in that same "negative" eating pattern.

But you can be better, because you are about to experience the powerful connection between food and performance, and in doing so, avoid that "negative" eating pattern.

By now you are probably wondering:

"How do I figure out which foods are right for my genetics?"

Simple, just complete the two-day Food Challenge outlined below.

When you are done, you will know how to monitor your body's response to food and which foods are more effective at energizing your body and mind and powering your soccer performance.

The Food Challenge

Your Food Challenge will involve eating one type of food one day, a different type of food on another day, and recording your body's response to both. A two-day commitment is all it takes.

The foods you will use for your Food Challenge are common, everyday foods. So you should have no trouble in obtaining them. However, you will need to be in control of your food during the two days of your Food Challenge.

Your two Food Challenge days do not have to be consecutive and should not be game days or days when a negative food effect could cause you any problems.

On your Food Challenge days:

- Stick closely to the program and do not mix in any other food or drink.
- Snack only if absolutely necessary.
- Drink only water unless otherwise instructed.
- Avoid taking supplements unless they are required for medical reasons, as they can affect your results.
- Do not skip a meal or any part of a meal.
- Maintain the same basic food portions if you need a second serving.

The goal is to learn which foods energize you and which don't. "Energized" means strong, steady energy. It does not mean "hyper" energy.

Your body thrives on steady energy. Big ups are usually followed by big downs, and that is not how your body performs at its best.

Before you begin you must:

- Have the correct foods available before starting your Food Challenge. If you eat in a cafeteria, check the weekly menu for a day when meals closest to those below are offered. They may not exactly match but do the best you can.
- Make two copies of the Meal Evaluation Form found in the Appendix of your *Soccer Nutrition Handbook*, one for each day of your Food Challenge. Do not start a Food Challenge day without having a Meal Evaluation Form in hand.

Day One Food Challenge Instructions

1. Choose your meals from the sample menu below. Each meal is based on the daily foods from Diet Plan #1, which can be found in the Appendix.

2. Apply the following portions when filling your plate:
   - Choose a protein portion the size of the palm of your hand
   - Choose a grain or pasta portion the size of your palm
   - Choose a vegetable portion twice the size of your palm

3. Eat slowly and do not overeat. Keep your meals relatively plain – minimize added salt, pepper and strong spices. Deep-fried foods are not allowed.

4. Avoid eating foods that do not appeal to you or that you know cause digestive problems or allergic reactions. You may substitute similar foods from Diet Plan #1 in the Appendix as needed.

5. On your Meal Evaluation Form, record what and how much you eat and drink at each meal. Then, one to two hours after each meal, record how you feel. It is important that you do this before eating any between-meal snacks.

Day One Food Challenge Sample Menu

<u>Breakfast - Day One</u> (choose one)

> Bowl of unsweetened cereal with 2% or skim milk or bowl of plain, unflavored oatmeal. If desired, sweeten with berries, banana or teaspoon of honey or sugar. Low-fat rice or almond milk may be used in place of 2% milk.

> Low-fat yogurt and/or several pieces of whole fruit (for example, melon, orange, grapefruit, berries or a mix of fruit with no added syrup); two pieces of whole grain toast or bagel with small amount of butter or virgin coconut oil.

> One cup of regular caffeinated coffee (adults only) with 2% milk, rice or almond milk (optional) and a teaspoon of

sugar (optional); a whole grain bagel or two pieces of whole grain toast with half a grapefruit or an orange, banana or other fruit. You may substitute herbal tea for the coffee or just have water.

Lunch - Day One (choose one)

Pasta with tomato sauce (no red meat or sausage in sauce); steamed vegetables; fruit such as an apple, banana, grapes, nectarine, orange, peach, pear, or plum.

Large garden salad with a hard-boiled egg or equivalent portion of chicken/turkey breast and vinaigrette dressing; a whole grain roll w/ small amount of butter (optional); fruit such as an apple, banana, grapes, nectarine, orange, peach, pear, or plum.

Chicken or turkey breast sandwich on whole grain bread; garden salad with vinaigrette dressing; fruit such as an apple, banana, grapes, nectarine, orange, peach, pear, or plum.

Dinner - Day One (choose one)

Grilled/broiled chicken/turkey breast; wild or brown rice; steamed vegetables such as squash, broccoli, carrot, pepper, Brussels sprouts or a garden salad with vinaigrette dressing.

Broiled white fish (cod, halibut, flounder, Mahi-mahi, trout, etc.); wild or brown rice; vegetables such as squash, broccoli, carrot, pepper, Brussels sprouts or a garden salad with vinaigrette dressing.

Grilled/broiled pork chop; baked potato or yam; vegetables such as squash, broccoli, carrot, pepper, Brussels sprouts or a garden salad with vinaigrette dressing.

Snacks - Day One (only if needed, record meal reaction before snacking)

- Carrot sticks
- Fruit (apple, banana, grapes, nectarine, orange, peach, pear, plum)

- Granola mix/bar (all natural)
- Low-fat unsweetened yogurt with fruit
- Sunflower seeds (modest portion)

Day Two Food Challenge Instructions

1. Choose your meals from the sample menu below. Each meal is based on the daily foods from Diet Plan #2, which can be found in the Appendix.

2. Apply the following portions when filling your plate:
   - Choose a protein portion the size of the palm of your hand.
   - Choose a grain portion the size of your palm.
   - Choose a vegetable portion twice the size of your palm.

3. Eat slowly and do not overeat. Keep your meals relatively plain – minimize added salt, pepper and strong spices. Deep-fried foods are not allowed

4. Avoid eating foods that do not appeal to you or that you know cause digestive problems or allergic reactions. You may substitute similar foods from Diet Plan #2 in the Appendix as needed.

5. On your Meal Evaluation Form, record what and how much you eat and drink at each meal. Then, one to two hours after each meal, record how you feel. It is important that you do this before eating a between-meal snack.

Day Two Food Challenge Sample Menu

<u>Breakfast – Day Two</u> (choose one)

Bacon and/or sausage and two eggs; one slice of whole grain toast or half a whole grain bagel with whole fat butter.

Steak and eggs; one slice of whole grain toast or half a whole grain bagel with whole fat butter.

Roast beef sandwich on whole grain bread (make the beef the majority of the sandwich, not the bread). This may not be considered a "normal" breakfast but it works well for this Food Challenge.

Lunch – Day Two (choose one)

Roast beef sandwich on whole grain bread (make the beef the majority of the sandwich, not the bread); spinach salad with vinaigrette dressing. Garnish with half or full avocado (optional).

Beef or buffalo burger (quarter to half pound) no bun or bread; raw, steamed or sautéed vegetables (asparagus, carrots, celery, cauliflower, corn, green beans, peas, spinach) or garden salad with vinaigrette dressing. Garnish with half or full avocado (optional).

Grilled or smoked wild salmon; raw, steamed or sautéed vegetables (asparagus, carrots, celery, cauliflower, corn, green beans, peas, spinach) or garden salad with vinaigrette dressing. Garnish with half or full avocado (optional).

Dinner – Day Two (choose one)

Chicken or turkey (dark – leg or thigh, not breast meat); raw, steamed or sautéed vegetables (asparagus, cauliflower, corn, green beans, peas); buttered wild or basmati rice (use virgin coconut oil instead of butter for non-dairy option).

Beef or buffalo steak with sautéed mushrooms (optional); raw, steamed or sautéed vegetables (asparagus, cauliflower, corn, green beans, peas, or spinach); buttered wild or basmati rice (use virgin coconut oil instead of butter for non-dairy option).

Grilled or broiled salmon; raw, steamed or sautéed vegetables (asparagus, cauliflower, corn, green beans, peas, or spinach); buttered wild or basmati rice (use coconut oil instead of butter for non-dairy option).

<u>Snacks – Day Two</u> (only if needed, record meal reaction before snacking)

- Apple slices with peanut or other nut butter
- Apple, berries, cherries, grapes, pear, peach (small amounts of fruit only)
- Celery sticks (with peanut or other nut butter)
- Almonds, peanuts, pecans, walnuts, pumpkin seeds

Evaluate Your Food Challenge Results

After completing your Food Challenge, compare the Day One and Day Two Meal Evaluation Forms.

If Day One stands out as the best day of food

Base your daily food selections and meals primarily from the foods listed on Diet Plan #1 (Appendix).

If Day Two stands out as the best day of food

Base your daily food selections and meals primarily from the foods listed on Diet Plan #2 (Appendix).

If both days worked well for you (Combo Diet)

Balance your daily food selections alternately between Diet Plan #1 and Diet Plan #2. For example, a red meat lunch (Diet Plan #2) can be followed by a white-fish dinner (Diet Plan #1).

The primary focus for the Combo Diet is alternating the type of protein between Diet Plans #1 and #2. This alternating pattern does not need to be meal by meal, but over the course of a few days, you should try to eat equally from both diet plans. The rest of the foods from Diet Plans #1 and #2 should be alternated as well, but if that becomes too difficult, they can be interchanged without causing major problems.

If neither diet plan seemed to work for you (rare but possible)

This may occur if you've been eating a high-sugar and/or high-caffeine and/or high-processed food diet and recently switched to whole foods and your body has not yet adapted.

Whether or not this is the case with you, the easiest solution is to continue to eat a low-sugar, low-caffeine, whole-food diet based on both diet plans and repeat the Food Challenge in two to four weeks.

Using Your Diet Plan

Now that you have identified the diet plan(s) that is right for you, it won't take long for you to learn your preferred foods. Here are a few suggestions:

- Make several copies of your diet plan(s).

- Post a copy in an easy-to-see place, such as on your refrigerator, and refer to it often while you prepare your meals.

- Carry a copy to the grocery store and to restaurants to help with food selection.

- Customize your diet plan by crossing off the foods that you absolutely don't like and won't eat, but keep in mind that tastes change and what you don't like today may one day become a favorite food.

How you implement your diet plan into your lifestyle is completely up to you. Keep your food selection process simple and stress-free.

One approach that works well is to "tilt" your food choices strongly toward the foods on your diet plan by following the 18-21 Rule. Make 18 of 21 meals each week healthy and from your diet plan.

As you progress, you will come to understand that learning how your body responds to food is an ongoing process, not an event. Take your time and enjoy the process.

Retesting

If at any time in the months following your Food Challenge you feel that your diet plan is no longer working for you, simply repeat the Food Challenge.

This change in dietary needs may occur as the body adjusts to eating foods that properly fuel it. It normally only takes one or two Food Challenges to dial-in a diet plan that works for you.

You should also keep in mind that changes in age, health, lifestyle, activities and stress can significantly affect your dietary needs. You may need to repeat the Food Challenge at a future date to meet those needs.

Menstrual Cycle (women only)

Hormonal changes during the phases of your menstrual cycle may alter your food needs. For most women this may only be a slight dietary change but, for some, a significant dietary change may be needed.

Common symptoms that may indicate the need to change your diet to match the cyclic nature of your menstrual cycle are:

- Strong cravings for red meat (Diet Plan #2) when you normally do well on white meat or fish (Diet Plan #1)
- Strong cravings for carbohydrates when you normally do well on a lower carbohydrate diet (Diet Plan #2)
- Your normally energizing foods make you feel tired or moody
- Extreme PMS symptoms

If any of these apply to you, you should start a monthly journal to monitor and record how you respond to your food during the different phases of your menstrual cycle. After a few months, you should see a pattern form.

Once you have identified your pattern, try altering the type of food you eat and monitor how your body responds to that food. For example, if you usually feel energized by white meat and white fish proteins (Diet Plan #1) and those stop working for you at a certain time of your menstrual cycle, try eating a small amount of red meat instead (Diet Plan #2) and monitor your body's response.

Sometimes it only takes a meal or two of eating your "cravings" to regain your dietary balance. Other times you may need to alter your intake for days or weeks. The only way to learn what works for you is to experiment and learn from what your body tells you.

After you recognize which foods are best during your menstrual cycle, continue to monitor your body's response as these dietary fluctuations can often diminish over time.

Step 4 Summary

- Learn your ideal foods by completing the Food Challenge and recording your body's response to each day of food on a Meal Evaluation Form.

- Once you know which Diet Plan(s) works best for you, choose the majority of the food you eat from that Diet Plan(s).

- If both Food Challenge days worked well for you, alternate food selections from Diet Plan #1 and #2 on a daily or meal by meal basis.

- Follow the 18-21 Rule – make 18 out of 21 meals each week healthy and from your Diet Plan.

- If neither Food Challenge day worked for you, continue to eat real (whole) food, limit sugar intake and eat equally from both diet plans for two to four weeks then repeat the Food Challenge.

- Continue to monitor your body's response to the food you eat and make adjustments as necessary. Repeat the Food Challenge anytime you feel that your Diet Plan is no longer working for you.

- Women— hormonal changes during your menstrual cycle may alter your food needs. Monitor and adjust as necessary.

STEP 5 - BALANCE YOUR PORTIONS

How well your meals provide you with lasting daily energy depends equally on two things:

- Eating the foods that work best for you – as determined by your Food Challenge.

- Eating the correct amount of protein, fat and carbohydrates at each meal.

The reason the amount of protein, fat and carbohydrates play such an important role is that they work together to provide your body with energy. Like teammates, each supports and depends on the other to get the job done.

For example, too much protein and too few carbohydrates at a meal can have the exact same effect as too many carbohydrates and too little protein – both can leave you low in energy and craving more food an hour or two after eating.

Get the amounts just right and you will have lasting energy and no food cravings.

Common Sources of Protein, Fat and Carbohydrates

Protein	Fat	Carbohydrate
Meat	Meat	Fruits
Poultry	Poultry	Vegetables
Seafood	Some fish (salmon, sardines)	Legumes
Eggs	Eggs	Grains
Nuts and Seeds	Butter, cheese, yogurt	Cereals
Legumes	Oils: fish, flax, olive, coconut	Breads
Dairy products	Nuts, seeds	Milk
Some whole grains	Avocados	Juice

The quickest and most effective way to determine how much protein, fat and carbohydrate you need at each meal is to experiment. You do not have to weigh or measure your food; measuring portions by eye is sufficient.

The amounts of protein and carbohydrates that work for you may also be different at breakfast than at lunch or dinner, or vice versa. It all depends on how your body uses its food energy and the demands you place on your body.

> **Note**
> While balancing your portions, it is best to avoid taking supplements unless they are required for medical reasons, as they can affect results.

Here are some starting points:

Diet Plan #1

- 60% carbohydrates (vegetables, fruits, grains)
- 40% protein and fat (eggs, light fish, light meat, nuts, seeds, dairy, virgin olive/coconut oil)

Diet Plan #2

- 40% carbohydrates (vegetables, fruits, grains)
- 60% protein and fat (eggs, oily fish, dark meat, nuts, seeds, dairy, virgin olive/coconut oil)

Diet Plan #1 and #2 Combination

- 50% carbohydrates (vegetables, fruits, grains)
- 50% protein and fat (eggs, fish, meat, nuts, seeds, dairy, virgin olive/coconut oil)

Start with breakfast and eat what you consider to be normal portions of protein and carbohydrates. Record your results on a Meal Evaluation Form. If the results are not positive – in particular you experience food cravings and/or an energy crash – increase the amount of protein and reduce the amount of carbohydrates at the next breakfast.

If you note an improvement, continue along those lines until you find the correct balance of protein and carbohydrate.

If increasing protein does not lead to improvement, go back to your starting point and reduce the amount of protein relative to carbohydrate until you find the optimum balance.

In some cases, you might feel best eating only protein for breakfast. If that is the case, continue to eat a protein-only breakfast until you begin to have negative reactions on your Meal Evaluation Form. Then add small amounts of carbohydrate, such as a half piece of toast or a small piece of fruit, to your breakfast until you find the correct balance.

Next, follow the same procedure with lunch, and then move on to dinner.

Do not try to figure out all your meals on the same days.

Take as many days as needed to figure out breakfast, and then move on to lunch and finally dinner.

By using this process, you will learn the powerful effect that food portions have on your daily energy, and you will be learning the life-long skill of how to "listen" to your body's response to food.

Step 5 Summary
- Use your Meal Evaluation Form to determine your ideal protein/fat to carbohydrate ratio at each meal.
- Ratios can be different at breakfast, lunch and dinner.
- Portion starting points:
    - Diet Plan #1: 60% carbohydrates, 40% protein/fat
    - Diet Plan #2: 40% carbohydrates, 60% protein/fat
    - Combo Diet Plan: 50% carbohydrates, 50% protein/fat

ADDITIONAL DIET PLAN GUIDELINES

Diet Plan #1

- Do not over eat high-starch carbohydrates (grains, baked goods, beans, potatoes and yams).
- Balance most of your meals with protein.
- Make vegetables and fruit your primary source of carbohydrate.
- Lean white/light meats, white fish, eggs, nuts, seeds and dairy are your primary sources of protein and fat.
- Fats such as olive oil, butter and coconut oil can be used in small quantities.
- Minimize foods with added sugars, sweet drinks and caffeine.

Diet Plan #2

- Eat protein at each meal but do not over eat protein.
- Best carbohydrate sources are vegetables and small portions of whole grains and fruit.
- Darker meats, oily fish, eggs, nuts, seeds and full-fat dairy should be your primary sources of protein and fat.
- Caution foods are high-starch foods like grains, baked goods, potatoes and yams, foods with added sugar, sweet drinks and caffeine.
- Fats such as olive oil, whole butter and coconut oil can be used in moderate quantities.
- Minimize foods with added sugars, sweet drinks and caffeine.

Combination Diet

- Follow the guidelines for each diet plan above.
- Eat equally from each diet plan over the course of a few days to a week paying particular attention to varying the type of protein you consume.
- Balance your meals with plenty of vegetables and moderate amounts of whole grains and fruit.
- Minimize foods with added sugars, sweet drinks and caffeine.

All Diet Plans

- Eat slowly to satisfaction and avoid overeating.
- Learn from what your body tells you about your food, both good and bad.
- The need for protein and fat can increase slightly during cold weather and decrease in warmer weather.
- Aging, growth, lifestyle changes, stress, illness and athletic challenges can affect your dietary needs.
- Between-meal food cravings are often best answered with a protein-based snack.

FROM FOOD TO FIELD: SENSING YOUR BODY'S RESPONSE

Now that you have a diet plan and your portions are balanced, you need to continue to develop the ability to sense how your body responds to food and drink. This is important because what you eat and when you eat it can dramatically affect your athletic performance.

Fortunately, it is an easy process because your body will provide feedback – all you need to do is learn to listen to your body. An effective way to do that is by using the Meal Evaluation Form daily for one week.

Choose a week when you will have at least four days of soccer practice or workouts. The goal is to monitor your body's response to your food and drink by observing your daily energy and athletic performance. The process takes only minutes each day.

Here's how:

- Make sufficient copies of the Meal Evaluation Form found in the Appendix.
- Record your daily food and drink intake and your body's response an hour or two after each meal.
- Record any snacks you consume and when you consume them.
- Record your hydration level prior to your practice, game or workout and how you felt during the activity.
- At the end of each day, rate your day of food.
- When you have completed your forms, evaluate your results:
    - Compare your overall day of food rating to your athletic performance.
    - Note which food and drink provided steady energy.
    - Note which food and drink crashed your energy.
    - Compare hydration levels to your athletic performance.
    - Note the amount of time between physical activity and your last meal or snack.

Learn from both good and bad results and make adjustments accordingly. You will need to experiment to determine what works best for you – paying particular attention to the timing of your meals prior to activity.

By the time you finish the week, listening to what your body is telling you about your food will be second nature and you will no longer need to use the forms. However, if you need more time or get off track with your food and performance, simply repeat this procedure. It's easy, effective, and it works!

OFF AND RUNNING

Congratulations on completing Section I. You now have the basic tools and knowledge to feed your body what it needs for optimum health and great performance both on and off the soccer field.

Soccer skills take time to learn and the same applies to nutrition skills. Make nutrition part of your soccer training and practice what you have learned until it becomes as natural as kicking a ball with your favorite foot.

Nutrition is an ongoing process, not an event. Continue to listen to your body's response to food and make adjustments as necessary.

If at any time you happen to get off track with your nutrition, just cut out the junk food and go back to feeding yourself simple, quality real foods and you will be back on track in no time. It's that simple.

> **The path you walk in the world of food will always be familiar if you let real foods be your map, and your body's response your compass.**

SECTION II

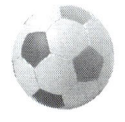

SOCCER SPECIFIC GUIDELINES

HYDRATION

The most important thing you can do as a soccer player is ensure you are properly hydrated before you step onto the field.

Adult soccer players typically lose about one quart (32 ounces) of water for each hour of playing time, and even more in hot, humid weather.

A reduction of just one to two percent of body weight due to water loss can significantly impair muscular performance.[1,2] Begin a game slightly dehydrated and you can easily be down two percent of your body weight by halftime.

For a 150-pound player, one to two percent of body weight is 1.5 to 3 pounds, which means that being under-hydrated by as little as a quart will impair performance.

In simple terms, if you enter a game even slightly dehydrated, your performance can suffer.

How Much to Drink

People sweat at different rates. A simple way to learn how much water you lose from exercise is to weigh yourself without clothes immediately before and after a workout. The difference is the net amount water weight lost during your workout.

Once you know how many pounds of water you have lost, re-hydrate by slowly drinking 16 to 24 ounces of fluid for each pound lost. If weighing yourself is not an option, a rule of thumb is to drink water frequently after your activity until your urine runs the color of pale lemonade or clear. Dark colored urine usually indicates dehydration.[3]

Individual variability (such as physical size) can affect your fluid needs, as can work out intensity and duration, humidity, altitude and temperature.

These hydration guidelines are provided as a starting point and should be modified as needed to accommodate your individual needs:[4,5,6,7]

- Hydrate daily. A baseline amount of water for a 150-pound athlete is two quarts (64 ounces) per day, not including exercise needs.
- Pregame or training:
  - Consume 16 to 24 ounces of water two to three hours before activity.
  - Consume 8 to 12 ounces of water 10 to 15 minutes before activity.
- During training:
  - Consume 8 to 12 ounces for each 15 minutes of activity.
  - If exercising longer than 90 minutes, drink 8 to 12 ounces of a "healthy" sports drink every 15 to 30 minutes.
- During halftime:
  - Drink fluid first, talk later. You have a limited time to rehydrate, use it wisely.
  - Drink small gulps of fluid until you feel satisfied but not overly full.
- Post-game/training:
  - Re-hydrate immediately after game or practice.
  - Drink 20 to 24 ounces of fluid for each pound of body weight lost during exercise, or until your urine runs clear or the color of pale lemonade.

Some additional considerations:

- The quality of your water matters. Choose filtered water whenever possible, cool during hot weather.
- Drink small amounts frequently rather than large amounts less frequently.
- If you feel thirsty the night before a morning game, you are probably not sufficiently hydrated.
- Over-hydration is rare but possible and can be hazardous. Listen to your thirst and consume fluid in quantities that approximate your sweat loss to avoid over-hydration.
- Avoid alcohol and caffeine or stimulant-laden drinks as they can dehydrate you.

Choosing the Right Water Bottle

A good way to ensure you always have pure water available is to carry a water bottle. It is also a great way to monitor how much you drink each day. The type of water bottle is important due to chemical contamination issues. Here are a few things to keep in mind when choosing a water bottle:

- Choose a water bottle with a wide mouth for easy cleaning.
- Glass bottles are contaminant free but are breakable. Foam/neoprene sleeves around a glass bottle can help with that problem. Glass-lined thermoses can keep liquids cold (or hot for cold-day games) but are heavy and bulky for the amount of fluid they contain.
- Food grade stainless steel water bottles are durable and considered to be contaminant free but some may impart a slight metallic taste to the water, particularly when warm.
- Aluminum water bottles typically have a lining on the inside of the bottle. Choose a brand that has a leach-free lining.

Avoid aluminum bottles if they are unlined or are not labeled as being leach-free.

Plastic water bottles are popular due to their durability and light weight. They are made from a variety of plastics, the type being indicated by the number (1 to 7) in the recycle triangle symbol on the bottom of the bottle.

The downside of plastic bottles is that some can leach health-damaging chemicals, such as BPA (Bisphenol A), into the water.[8]

The effects of BPA are still being studied, but there is evidence that it may cause developmental problems in the brains and hormonal systems of fetuses and children, and may increase the risk of certain cancers, heart disease and diabetes.[9,10,11]

Until more research is completed, it is best to limit your exposure to these chemicals.

The following general guidelines can help in that regard:

- If you taste plastic when you drink from your water bottle, get a different bottle.
- Only use plastic water bottles that are BPA-free.
- #1 PET (polyethylene terephthalate), #2 HDPE (high density polyethylene), #4 LDPE (low density polyethylene), #5 PP (polypropylene) and some #7 (other) products are generally considered to be safe in a BPA-free version.
- #3 (PVC) and #6 (styrene) should be avoided.

Health-wise, the best water bottles are glass and stainless steel. Contaminant-free plastic and leach-free lined aluminum bottles are also an acceptable option.

Sports Drinks versus Water

Water is usually sufficient for a well-fed, well-conditioned soccer player participating in one game or practice per day in average temperatures.

Multiple sessions per day of intense exercise on hot, humid days can drain the body of carbohydrates and electrolytes such as magnesium, potassium, sodium and chloride.

Sports drinks are designed to replenish carbohydrates and electrolytes both during and after intense exercise that lasts longer than 60 to 90 minutes.[12,13]

Unless playing in extreme temperatures or conditions or playing multiple games in one day, the duration and intensity of children's soccer games is rarely enough to warrant the use of sport drinks.

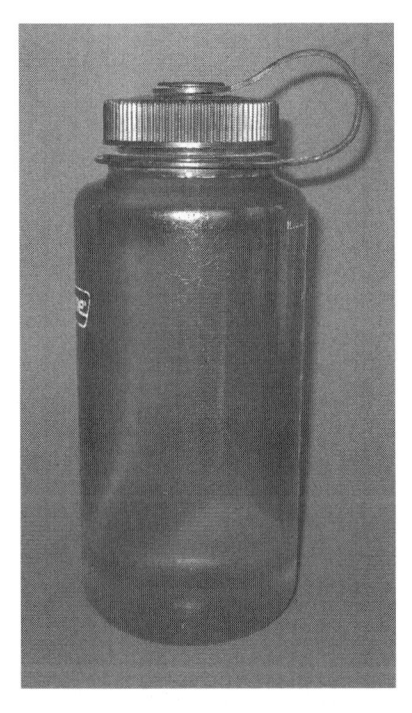

This wide-mouth, quart-sized, BPA-free, plastic water bottle is durable, easy to clean and large enough to get you through most soccer games.

In most soccer situations, young players should just drink water.

The high levels of sugar and added ingredients such as artificial flavors, colors and sweeteners in most sports drinks make them unhealthy on a fundamental level. Thus, sport drinks should only be used for their intended purpose and should not be consumed as a casual, daily beverage as many athletes mistakenly do.

The best health-promoting casual beverage is pure water.

To learn if sports drinks work for you, experiment during training and focus on how your body responds. Compare the results to how you feel if you only drink water. You may find, as many do, that you do equally well or even better with water.

Do not get caught up in the advertising hype of sports drink manufacturers. Despite their claims, there is no miracle in a bottle.

Sport Drink Quality

The sugar content, the type of sugar, artificial colors, flavors and sweeteners and electrolyte content all factor into the quality of a sports drink.

Here are some guidelines for choosing a "healthier" sports drink:

- Avoid those containing high fructose corn syrup (HFCS). The growing controversy concerning the possible negative health effects of HFCS is enough to warrant avoiding it. HFCS may also be listed in the ingredients as "glucose-fructose syrup."

- Avoid sports drinks that contain artificial colors and flavors and artificial sweeteners (see Artificial Sweeteners in Section I).

- Choose drinks that have a higher electrolyte and vitamin content.

- Avoid drinks that contain stimulants such as caffeine and Guarana – a form of caffeine from a South American berry. Common side effects of these stimulants often include:

    o   Anxiety

    o   Heart palpitations

- Hyperactivity
- Insomnia
- Trembling
- Frequent urination

None of these side effects benefit soccer performance.

Much has been written about sport drinks with added protein improving on-field performance. Some studies support that claim, many do not.

A more appropriate use of this type of sports drink may be as a post-workout recovery drink, although the unhealthy nature of some of the ingredients often used in these products makes real food and pure water a better choice.

Make Your Own Sports Drink

Many athletes make their own sports drink. By doing so they control the quality of the ingredients and can adjust the mix to meet their individual needs. It is also much less expensive than buying a commercial product.

The carbohydrate content should be approximately 6 percent, which equates to 14 grams of carbohydrate per 8 ounces of water, or 56 grams per quart. Higher amounts of carbohydrate can cause stomach upset during exercise.

Here is a quick and easy sport drink recipe that makes one quart:

- 1/2 quart pure organic fruit juice (no added sugar)
- 1/2 quart water
- 1/8 to 1/4 teaspoon sea salt

You may need to adjust the amount of juice to obtain 6 percent carbohydrate content.

This recipe provides approximately 60 to 120 mg of sodium per 8-ounce serving depending on the type of sea salt used.

GAME DAY NUTRITION

Perhaps the most common question soccer players ask is: "What should I eat on game day?"

Often, the thinking behind this question is that by eating a special meal on game day, you will somehow boost your performance

**Performance nutrition
is not a one-day or one-meal event.**

It is a daily activity, all year long. It is about nourishing your body well over a significant period of time so that each of your many trillion cells can perform its designed function to make you strong, fit and as clear thinking as possible.

That is not to say that what you eat will not affect how you perform on game day. It can. Wash down four slices of spicy pizza with a 24-ounce soda an hour before kick-off and your body will need a digestive miracle to avoid vomiting during the first half.

However, if you eat well on a daily basis and take the time to learn how your body responds to your food, you will already know exactly what to eat on game day.

Here are a few suggestions for game day nutrition:

- Eat your ideal foods from your Diet Plan in the correct proportions during the days leading up to your game. This is the best way to get nutritionally ready to play. The same approach applies for your pregame meal.

- Hydrate the day before and the day of the game by drinking small quantities of water often (see Hydration in Section II).

- For morning games, get to bed early enough the night before to get a full night's rest and allow at least two hours to digest your breakfast.

- Choose non-spicy, easily-digested foods for your pregame meal. Nerves tend to be high on game day and dropping spicy food into an already nervous stomach is a recipe for trouble. Avoid these foods for your pregame meal:
    - Deep-fried foods (chicken, French fries, etc.)
    - Ice cream/milk shakes
    - Raw onions, broccoli and cabbage
    - Beans (in large amounts)
    - Grapefruit and large amounts of citrus juice
    - Chocolate (brownies, etc.)
    - Hot dogs, bratwurst, sausage, bacon

Practice eating a pre-game meal before a few of your training sessions to learn which foods work best for you and how long you need to digest them. That way when game day arrives, you will know exactly how much of which foods to consume.

Plan your game day in advance. Whenever possible, pack your own pregame meal and snacks and eat the quantity of food that you know works for you. Your body will do better slightly hungry than stuffed full.

Should You Carbohydrate Load?

Carbohydrate loading was introduced some forty years ago as a way for endurance athletes to boost the amount of energy stored in their muscles prior to a long distance race.

In simple terms, carbohydrate loading is done by reducing your carbohydrate intake a week in advance of an event and then increasing your carbohydrate intake during the three to four days leading up the event. At the same time, you taper physical activity to almost zero as you near your event.

While carbohydrate loading may benefit some marathoners and endurance athletes, the practice is impractical and often unwise for soccer players. Here are a few reasons why:

- Genetics – some athletes do not do well on a higher carbohydrate diet, even for one or two meals. For them, carbohydrate loading leads to blood sugar imbalances and energy crashes.

- Gender – the food needs of women can change significantly with the phase of their menstrual cycle. Eating a lot of carbohydrates at a time when they are not what the body needs can lead to reduced energy production and impaired athletic performance.

- Timing – soccer seasons are full of games and training sessions. Rarely is there a full week in which to prepare your body for one game.

A far more practical and workable approach is to eat well on a daily basis and maintain intake of the foods that best fuel your body in the correct proportions as you learned in Section I.

By doing so, you will maintain energy reserves in your muscles and not have to worry about timing and possible blood sugar crashes.

Depending on your individual needs, you may choose to slightly increase your carbohydrate intake the day or night before game day to ensure your muscles are "topped off." For instance, you may choose to eat a second portion of whole grain rice or pasta with your meals the day before a big game.

This may work for you but you should try it in a practice situation first. The middle of a game is not the time to learn that it doesn't work for you.

Our experience at Nutrition Coaches, LLC has shown that in most soccer situations, the practice of carbohydrate loading is impractical and often does more harm than good.

Recovery Food and Drink

When it comes to post-game or post-practice food and drink, there is a lot of hype from sport drink and energy bar manufacturers.

According to them, if you even come close to breaking a sweat during exercise, you immediately become electrolyte-deprived, vitamin-starved and horribly dehydrated. In other words, use their product or you will fail as an athlete.

It's a good sales pitch, but considering that humans have been performing incredible feats of athleticism for thousands of years without those products, clearly there is a disconnect somewhere.

When you exercise, you deplete energy reserves and break down muscle tissue. To recharge your body's energy and help rebuild your muscles, it makes sense to eat carbohydrates and a small amount of protein after you work out. These are called recovery foods.

However, you don't need to eat recovery food after every workout. The intensity and duration of your workout determines your recovery food needs. The harder and longer you work out, the more recovery foods can help.

For example:

- If you endure a hard training session in the morning and will be training again later that day, you should eat something soon after your first session to help your body recover before the second session.

- If you are a substitute player and only play half a game, the need for recovery foods is minimal.

How soon you need to recover should also play a role in deciding if you need recovery foods. Between a game Sunday morning and practice Tuesday afternoon is plenty of time for your body to fully recover with normal healthy meals and proper hydration.

Here are some basic guidelines concerning recovery foods:

- Plan your day so your recovery food is available after a hard workout or game.
- Experiment after practice to learn which foods your body "likes" and how much of those foods to eat. Your individual needs can depend on your overall nutritional wellness, level of physical fitness, amount of exertion, how much you sweat, etc.
- Try to eat your chosen recovery food within 30 minutes of finishing a hard workout, particularly if you next meal is a couple of hours away. If your next meal is within an hour, that can be your recovery food.
- When possible, choose real food over less healthy sport drinks and energy bars. Here are a few recovery food examples:
    - Bagel with peanut butter or other nut butter
    - Fruit juice or several pieces of fruit and a handful of nuts
    - Trail mix containing dried fruit and nuts
    - Half of a chicken, turkey or ham sandwich and some fruit
    - Healthy granola bar with nut butter for protein
    - Fruit smoothie with protein powder
    - Protein bar and sports drink (convenient but often not as healthy)
- Avoid large amounts of high-fat and protein-dense foods as they digest slowly. The goal is to eat nutritious foods that digest quickly for rapid energy and nutrient replacement.

- If you have difficulty eating immediately after working out, your best option might be a sports drink that contains protein or a liquid protein or meal replacement shake.

Recovery food or not, be sure to hydrate properly after all workouts and games.

How much recovery food you need immediately after a hard workout is unique to you. At Nutrition Coaches, LLC we suggest the following within 30 minutes of finishing a strenuous soccer game:

- Carbohydrates: Consume the same number of grams of carbohydrate as half your body weight in pounds. Example: a 150-pound athlete needs about 75 grams of carbohydrate.

- Protein: Consume the same number of grams of protein as 1/10th your body weight in pounds. Example: a 150-pound athlete needs about 15 grams of protein.

A large, whole-grain bagel contains about 60 grams of carbohydrate and 5 grams of protein. Add 6 grams of carbohydrate and 8 grams of protein from 2 tablespoons of peanut butter and the total is close enough to be an acceptable post-game snack for a 150-pound player.

When it comes to recovery foods, keep it simple and understand that there are no exact rules to follow – close is good enough and whatever works best for you is what you should do.

Even with no recovery food after a game or tough practice your body will recover just fine if you eat normal, healthy meals and hydrate properly soon after playing. It may just take a few extra hours to get there.

Did You Know?
1 ounce of meat contains approximately 8 grams of protein.

3 ounces of meat is about the size of a deck of cards.

TOURNAMENT PLAY

Soccer tournaments are a physical, mental and a nutritional challenge. Games are often spaced only hours apart or sometimes back to back, and you can play three, one-hour games in a day for two or three days in a row. The physical demands of that kind of schedule are intense.

Tournament games are more often decided by mental mistakes rather than physical ones, and experienced players know that fatigue leads to mental mistakes.

Keeping yourself properly fueled can help reduce mental mistakes. Here are a few simple guidelines to get you in nutritional shape for tournament play:

Before the Tournament

- Eat your ideal foods from your Diet Plan in the correct proportions during the week leading up to your tournament to get yourself nutritionally fit.

- Hydrate the day before the tournament by drinking small quantities of water throughout the day. How much water you drink that day will vary according to your starting level of hydration, physical size, activity level, and how much liquid is provided by your food. Drink until you feel satisfied.

- It can take 24 hours to properly hydrate your body so if you feel a strong thirst the night before an early game, you are probably not well hydrated.

- Go to bed early enough the night before the tournament to get a full night's rest and allow at least two hours before game time to digest your favorite pre-game breakfast.

- Sleeping in and skipping the first meal of the day can create a nutritional deficit that can ruin your on-field performance.

- Prior to the tournament, complete a quick online search to find restaurants and supermarkets near the tournament fields to make finding and buying supplies easier. Supermarkets can provide a healthier and less expensive alternative to eating in restaurants.
- Plan ahead so you have food and drink available at the field. If you have to wait for someone else to go pick something up, you may miss the opportunity to be nutritionally ready for the next game.

During the Tournament
One Hour Between Games

- Drink fluid immediately after the first game.
- Here are a few options to consider should you feel the need for a snack:
    - A small portion of fruit from your Diet Plan – half a banana, small plum, grapes, etc.
    - A small portion of bagel or bread with or without peanut or other nut butter.
    - Dried fruit can also work when used in quantities similar to what you would eat in the non-dried form.
    - Use a sports drink only if you know it works for you. Your own mix is preferable.
- If you eat any solid food, eat it immediately after the game you just played and chew it thoroughly to help your digestive system process it more efficiently.
- Do not overeat between games. Your body will do better slightly hungry than on a full stomach.

Several Hours Between Games

- Eat a small portion of fruit after the game you just played and immediately begin rehydrating.

- Eat a "between-game" meal, allowing enough time to digest the food before your next game. Two hours is an average time but you may need more or slightly less depending on how much and what you eat.
- Your between-game meal should consist of a lean protein such as turkey, beef or chicken (pick from your Diet Plan) and relatively high content of carbohydrates.
- A whole or half sandwich on whole-grain bread and some whole fruit is often a good choice.
- Avoid heavy, greasy, spicy and hard-to-digest foods:
    o Deep-fried foods (chicken, French fries, etc.)
    o Ice cream/milk shakes
    o Raw onions, broccoli and cabbage
    o Beans (in large amounts)
    o Grapefruit and large amounts of citrus juice
    o Chocolate (brownies, etc.)
    o Hot dogs, bratwurst, sausage, bacon
- Sip water regularly between games. Use a sports drink only if you know it works for you.

After the Last Game of the Day

- Immediately begin to rehydrate and within 30 minutes eat some carbohydrates and a small amount of protein.
- An example is a bagel with peanut butter. Some fruit and a small handful of nuts is another. A protein-fruit smoothie is also a good choice.
- Within an hour or two, eat a normal meal. This will give your body what it needs to replenish depleted energy and speed muscle recovery.

- If you sweat excessively during the tournament, adding a little extra salt to your food can help replace the sodium lost through sweating.

- Continue to hydrate throughout the evening. Clear or pale lemonade-colored urine indicates you are properly rehydrating.

Preparation is the key to doing well in a tournament. Being both physically and nutritionally fit on your way into a tournament will help you play your best throughout the tournament.

SURVIVING A FAST-FOOD SITUATION

You're traveling with your team to play a game in the middle of the afternoon. The coach decides to stop for a team lunch. Unfortunately, the only option is a fast-food burger joint.

The meat is factory farmed and greasy, the hamburger buns are white bread, not whole grain, much of the food is deep-fried and the beverages are laden with sugar or artificial sweeteners.

This scenario gets played out by high school and college teams across the country, and even in the higher ranks of play. Is a fast-food, pre-game meal a game changer? It certainly can be if you choose the wrong foods.

Despite the poorer quality of food typically available, you can do "okay" at most fast-food restaurants. If you eat well on a daily basis, your body can handle the occasional not-so-desirable meal.

Here are a few things to keep in mind to make the best of a fast-food situation:

- Avoid eating it! If possible, prepare your game-day, travel-food before you get on the road. Bring food with you that you know works for you.

- Examples might be fruit, a mix of nuts and dried fruit or make a sandwich and carry it in a small, soft-sided cooler.

That way, if the option the coach chooses for the team pre-game meal doesn't work for you, you will be prepared.

- If you don't remember to bring food, your next step is to make intelligent choices.

- Avoid spicy, heavy, greasy and deep-fried foods. Burping up pepperoni pizza while sprinting down the field won't win games.

- Choose clean and lean sources of nutrition that are closest to foods from your Diet Plan, and maintain your ideal protein and fat to carbohydrate ratio as best you can. When choosing meats, choose grilled or baked over deep-fried.

- Bring your own source of "clean" water whenever possible. Tap water quality can vary dramatically from one location to the next – even from one county to the next – and a water-borne microbe your digestive system hasn't seen before can quickly cause significant gastric disturbance.

- Avoid sweet drinks or those that contain artificial sweeteners – soda, milkshakes, fruit drinks, lemonade, energy drinks, sweet teas and coffee drinks are best avoided.

Just because a 22-ounce soda is part of combo-meal #6 doesn't mean you have to drink it. Drink small amounts of water with your meals.

- Experiment on practice days to learn which pre-game foods work best for you and when to consume them relative to game time. Stick to what works for you even if it means not participating in a team pre-game food activity.

- If you know that you do better eating a small piece of fruit an hour before you play, make sure you have that fruit available an hour before you play.
- If before a game a teammate, parent or coach tells you to eat or drink some "super-energy" something or other that you have never tried before, politely decline it.

Game day is not experiment day. Stick with what you know works for you.

There are numerous types of fast food restaurants – sub sandwich shops, hamburger joints, fried chicken places, pizza and to-go Asian-food restaurants to name a few. Most are inexpensive, convenient, and can quickly serve a team with mass-produced food.

The type of fast-food restaurant your coach chooses can make a big difference, but once inside the choices you make are even more important.

The best fast-food restaurants for a team on the road have enough variety to satisfy everyone in the group. This means a place that serves several different types of lean protein, both light and dark, and where vegetables and fruit are also available.

Sandwich shops are often a good choice as most offer a variety of lean protein, vegetable toppings and whole grain breads. Restaurants with salad bars are also good choices.

As a soccer player, you face difficult situations in every game. Fast food on the road is merely an off-field situation that is easily handled by preparing in advance and making smart food choices.

In summary:
- Understand that the quality of fast-food may not be great but if you eat well on a regular basis, your body can handle it.
- Avoid spicy, heavy, greasy and deep-fried foods.
- Avoid sweet drinks. Drink small amounts of water with your meal.
- Whenever possible, bring foods that you know work as your pregame meal.
- Choose foods as close as possible to those from your Diet Plan, particularly the type of protein.
- Eat the quantity of food that you know works for you.
- Maintain the protein and fat to carbohydrate ratio that works for you.
- Eat what you know works for you on game day – do not experiment.

GETTING THE MOST FROM YOUR CAFETERIA

As a soccer player in high school or college, cafeteria food may be your primary source of nutrition. If so, what you choose to eat and drink in that setting can make a big difference in how you feel and play.

College freshman are noted for putting on the "freshman 15" – the 15 pounds of body fat that many accumulate during their first year at school. This is usually the result of making poor food choices in an all-you-can-eat cafeteria setting.

Many soccer players also struggle with health and body fat issues for the same reason. Cafeterias offer many different foods that vary greatly in quality. This can make choosing which and how much food to eat a nutritional challenge.

When eating in a cafeteria, follow your Diet Plan as much as possible and adopt a "do the best you can" attitude.

Here are some guidelines to help you make good food decisions in your cafeteria:

- Follow the 18-21 Rule – make 18 out of 21 meals each week healthy.

- As best you can, maintain a balance in each meal: a good starting point is to make 1/4 of your meal protein, 1/4 of your meal whole grain, 1/2 of your meal vegetables (see Balance Your Portions in Section I).

- Eat slowly and finish when slightly less than full. The temptation of "all you can eat" can easily lead to overeating and body fat accumulation.

- Arrive early to the cafeteria as the best foods are often prepared and served first.

- Supplement cafeteria food with food you buy from a grocery store. For example, keep a supply of nuts/fruits/veggies around for snacks.

- Minimize sugary foods and drinks such as cakes, cookies, ice cream, soda, sweet teas, juice, sport drinks, etc. Cafeterias provide many of these foods and drinks, and it is easy to get into a habit of eating a sweet treat and drinking a sweet drink at every meal.

- Drink water, filtered if possible. This is your best choice for most meals. Herbal tea can be a flavorful change. Most fruit juice is loaded with added sugar – a good rule to follow is that if you want the juice, eat the whole fruit.

The College Cafeteria

Problem: Your late afternoon soccer practice doesn't end in time for you to make it to the cafeteria for dinner before it closes.

Solution: Have a supply of healthy food in your dorm room or apartment so you won't be stuck eating microwave popcorn, delivery pizza or vending machine food for dinner.

- Organic milk is an okay choice if you are not allergic to or intolerant of dairy. However, it is rare to find organic milk in a cafeteria. Therefore, do not over-consume cafeteria milk. And remember, milk should be treated as a food, not a thirst-quenching beverage.

- Minimize deep-fried foods such as deep-fried chicken and fish. If you must eat it, strip off the outer layer of breading and skin and eat the meat underneath. By doing so you will be reducing the amount of unhealthy fat from the deep frying process.

- Pizza and pasta are common cafeteria foods and should be eaten only occasionally. In addition to being remarkably fattening, pizza often contains a great deal of "unhealthy" fat, sugar and low quality protein. If you eat pasta, keep the portion reasonable in size (palm of hand) and add some protein.

- Tomato-based sauces and ketchup usually contain large amounts of sugar. Use just enough to add flavor.

- Eat lean protein when it is served. Examples: eggs (from shell is preferable to powdered), lean beef, lean pork, chicken, turkey, etc. Avoid deep-fried foods.

- Most cafeterias have a salad bar. Eat from that at least once per day to fill up on fresh vegetables. Two times per day is better.

- Choose whole fruit over canned fruit. Canned fruit often is loaded with added sugar/syrup and there may be issues with BPA contamination from the lining of the can (see Produce in Section VI).

- Choose whole grain breads over white breads.

- Cooked whole grains are not common in cafeterias. Instant white rice is very common but not very nutritious. Limit portions of white rice and combine with beans or a stir-fry. Choose wild or brown rice when available.

- Many cafeteria vegetables are canned and over-cooked. Still, they will provide some nutrients and fiber to aid with digestion and elimination. Many cooked vegetables are seasoned with butter, so if you have a food allergy or sensitivity to dairy, keep that in mind.

- Eat a non-sweet breakfast whenever possible. Breakfast tends to be the least healthy meal in cafeterias. Cereal, low quality or pre-packaged eggs, processed meats like sausage or bacon, waffles, pancakes and sweetened oatmeal are commonly served.

  o You will probably need to supplement with your own food from outside the cafeteria to get a healthy breakfast. Some cafeterias offer omelets, which can be a good choice if made with vegetables.

  o Consume eggs no more than 3 to 4 times per week to avoid developing an egg-allergy issue.

  o Unflavored oatmeal usually has less sugar than flavored types. To make it more flavorful, add fruit and nuts.

  o Unsweetened, whole-grain breakfast cereals are nutritionally better than their sweetened counterparts.

In summary, choose foods that have been processed and sweetened the least and you will be making the best of your cafeteria situation.

SECTION III

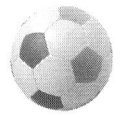

SUPPLEMENTS, SHAKES, BARS AND GOO

Supplements

There are many nutrients needed by the human body, and like players on a good team, they work together in harmony. Just as one player cannot succeed alone on a soccer field, believing that one nutrient will somehow boost performance and health without considering the interactions and contributions of all the others is flawed thinking.

For example, calcium plays a vital role in bone health, and people with weak bones often take a calcium supplement to build bone strength.

However, the absorption and utilization of calcium depends strongly on magnesium, phosphorous, copper, sodium, potassium and vitamin D. A deficiency in one or more of those can render calcium supplementation ineffective.

Real, whole foods naturally provide nutrients in balanced amounts, making them essential to good health and top athletic performance. The nutrient deficiency or imbalanced nutrient content of industrial foods can make them problematic.

Supplements are designed to complement a healthy diet, not to compensate for unhealthy eating. Adding a vitamin pill to a meal of French fries, cookies and soda does not make it healthy.

Do You Need To Take Nutritional Supplements?

If you eat quality whole foods every day, the answer to that question would likely be no. But that is often not the case. Therefore, to ensure a balanced nutrient intake, some supplementation is recommended.

That does not mean you need to take every supplement under the sun. More is not better, and too many can have serious negative health consequences.

The general consensus is that vitamin supplements can improve sport performance only in athletes who are vitamin deficient.[1,2] Therefore, the primary goal of nutrient supplementation is to prevent or correct nutrient deficiency.

> **What is RDA?**
> The Recommended Dietary Allowance (RDA) is the average daily amount of a nutrient considered adequate to meet the known nutrient needs of practically all healthy people.
> The purpose of this standard is prevention of nutrient deficiency disease, not health optimization.

The best way to accomplish this is to first establish a healthy eating routine by following your diet plan and balancing your portions, and then gradually add in supplements as needed.

If you have a known nutrient deficiency or nutrient-related illness, you should consult with your healthcare provider concerning specific supplement needs.

Choosing Quality Supplements

Walk into a store that sells supplements and you are likely to see hundreds if not thousands of bottles of pills, powders and liquids, each with their own formulation and claims of being the best.

If you are not knowledgeable about supplements, you can spend a small fortune trying supplement after supplement and chasing the latest media buzzword or "magic bullet" without attaining any appreciable gains in health.

Here are some guidelines to make supplement selection easier:

Where to buy?

- Choose stores that specialize in health products. Department, grocery and drug stores tend to offer lower quality supplements.
- Online suppliers often offer a wider variety and lower price than local stores.

What to buy?

- Food-based supplements – nutrients labeled "made from whole food" are preferable to synthetic versions derived from chemicals and petroleum products.
- Multi-formulas are easier and less expensive than creating your own mix of vitamins and minerals. The exception would be to treat a specific nutrient deficiency or to avoid sensitivity to a particular ingredient.
- Be cautious of formulas that contain herbs. Herbs can have powerful effects and many should not be taken on a long term basis.

Cost and Quality

- Quality supplements can be expensive. If cost is a consideration, take a quality supplement every other day rather than a lesser-quality daily.
- Higher quality supplements tend to be more bio-available (more easily absorbed by your body) – more of low-quality supplements may end up in your toilet than in you.
- Choose hypo-allergenic products to reduce the chance of a sensitivity reaction.
- Store sales clerks may or may not be well informed about supplements. For more information, ask the person who buys supplements for the store or call the supplement company directly.

- Choose supplements labeled "contaminant free" whenever possible.

> **Common Forms of Nutrient Measure**
>
> Milligram (mg) = 1/1,000 of a gram (28,350 mg per ounce)
>
> Microgram (mcg) = 1/1,000 of a milligram
>
> International Unit (IU), a measure of the amount of a substance based on its biological activity or effect. The precise definition of one IU differs from substance to substance. For example, one IU of vitamin E does not contain the same number of milligrams as one IU of vitamin A.

What Form?

- Capsules or tablets are more convenient than liquids and powders.
- Divided doses are preferred to a once-a-day mega-dose.
- Be wary of artificial sweeteners or flavors in liquid supplements.
- Tablet or capsule dissolvability is important. To test, put one in a in a glass of body-temperature water and wait one hour. If it hasn't mostly dissolved, you would do well to choose a different brand.

When to take?

- Unless otherwise directed, take supplements with meals. Your body expects nutrients to come from food, not from an empty stomach.
- When taking supplements, you should monitor your body's reaction in the same way that you do with your food. Supplements can be person specific, and you may need to try several brands before you find one that works well for you.

Which Supplements Should You Take?

The following recommendations are designed to support athletic performance and address some nutrient deficiencies common to many athletes:

- Multi-vitamin / mineral (MVM) daily supplement
- Vitamin C
- Vitamin D – only if a blood test reveals a deficiency, and then only under the supervision of a healthcare provider

Each of these supplements is discussed in detail below.

In addition, consuming a balance of essential fats is highly recommended for athletes. They play a powerful role in performance, recovery and injury healing. As essential fats are primarily food-sourced, they are discussed later in Section V.

CAUTION!	To prevent drug interactions and/or toxicity issues, always consult with your healthcare provider before taking any nutritional supplements.

What's in a Nutritional Supplement?

Supplements may contain some or all of the following:

Vitamins:
- Organic nutrients required in tiny amounts to promote growth, reproduction, body maintenance and health
- Can be destroyed by light, exposure to oxygen or high temperatures (pasteurization or cooking)
- Two forms are:
    o Water soluble: B and C vitamins
    o Fat soluble: Vitamins A, D, E and K (can be toxic in excess)

Minerals:
- Inorganic elements that are not affected by heat, light or oxygen
- Play a vital role in every body function including fluid balance, bone structure, muscle function, nerve function, etc.

- Major Minerals: calcium, magnesium, potassium, sodium, chloride, phosphorus and sulfur
- Trace Minerals: iron, zinc, iodine, selenium, copper, manganese, fluoride, chromium molybdenum and others

Amino Acids:
- The building blocks of body proteins
- Food protein is broken down in the digestive tract into amino acids, which are then absorbed and used by your cells to make thousands of different body proteins
- There are twenty common amino acids, nine of which the body cannot make and therefore must be supplied by food

Phytochemicals:
- Hundreds of plant compounds such as beta carotene, lutein, and lycopene
- In food they impart taste, color, aromas, and other characteristics
- In your body they act as antioxidants, mimic hormones and fight disease

Antioxidants:
- Enzymes and molecules that work to neutralize tissue-damage
- Common examples are vitamins (C and E), minerals, and many phytochemicals

Herbs:
- Plants and plant extracts
- Used primarily for treating specific health conditions or deficiencies

General Recommendations

Multi-Vitamin/Mineral

Multivitamin/mineral (MVM) supplements are a convenient way to get a balanced combination of nutrients in a single product.

Avoid MVM formulas that contain iron unless you have been diagnosed as iron deficient or have a history of iron deficiency. Always seek advice of your healthcare provider when considering iron supplementation.

Chewable MVM formulas often lack certain bad-tasting but beneficial nutrients and may contain artificial sweeteners.

Vitamin C

Humans are one of the few mammals on Earth that do not make their own vitamin C (ascorbic acid). Consequently, vitamin C must come from our diet.

Some of the many health benefits associated with vitamin C are:

- Growth and repair of tissues throughout the body such as skin, tendons, ligaments, and blood vessels – injury recovery
- Strong immune system function
- Healthy cartilage, bones and teeth
- Reduces inflammation – for example, from excess exercise
- Powerful antioxidant properties that combat the development of cancer, heart disease and arthritis
- Reduces the effects of air pollution and chemicals

> **Fortified Foods**
> Some food products, such as breakfast cereals, are heavily fortified with vitamins and minerals.
> If you eat those products, make sure you are not getting too much in the way of supplements if you also take a multi-vitamin/mineral supplement.

A lack of vitamin C can lead to:

- Gum bleeding
- Slow injury healing
- Easy bruising and nosebleeds
- Swollen and painful joints
- Anemia / fatigue
- Dry skin and hair
- Decreased ability to fight infection
- Possible weight gain due to slowed metabolism

A complete lack of vitamin C in the diet will eventually result in death from scurvy. The current RDA (Recommended Dietary Allowance) for vitamin C is:

RECOMMENDED DIETARY ALLOWANCE FOR VITAMIN C

Age	Male	Female
14-18	75 mg per day	65 mg per day
Over 18	90 mg per day	75 mg per day

Many health professionals consider these levels to be completely inadequate, especially when compared to the much larger amounts produced by other mammals. For example, a man-sized goat would make 13 grams (13,000 mg) of vitamin C per day.[3]

Extensive study has shown that vitamin C supplementation in a healthy general adult population is safe up to 2,000 mg (2 grams) per day on a long term basis.[4]

Much higher levels of vitamin C have been used therapeutically with no significant side effects.[5]

Vitamin C in Your Multi

If your multi-vitamin/mineral supplement provides a high level of vitamin C, additional vitamin C supplementation may not be needed. Most do not.

Nutrition Coaches, LLC recommends regular consumption of vitamin C rich foods and a daily vitamin C supplement. Common foods high in vitamin C are:

- Citrus fruits
- Strawberries
- Broccoli
- Leafy greens
- Tomatoes
- Potatoes
- Peppers

When starting vitamin C supplementation, increase your dosage gradually over the course of one to two weeks. If you experience loose stools or gastric disturbance, reduce your dosage.

RECOMMENDED VITAMIN C SUPPLEMENTATION

Age	Male and Female
Under 10 years	Consult with healthcare provider
10 -14 years	500 mg once or twice daily
Over 14 years	1,000 mg (1 gram) once or twice daily

If you decide to stop taking vitamin C, gradually reduce your consumption to avoid immune system disruption.

Buffered forms of vitamin C are available for those who cannot tolerate the acidity of regular ascorbic acid. Both buffered and non-buffered forms of vitamin C seem to work equally well.

CAUTION!	If you have Hemochromatosis (excess iron), consult with your healthcare provider as vitamin C supplements can boost iron absorption and cause iron toxicity.

Vitamin D

Your body makes vitamin D when your skin is exposed to sunlight. You can also get limited amounts from the food you eat.

It is estimated that 40 to 50 percent of the children and young adults in the United States are vitamin D deficient, primarily due to lack of exposure to sunlight and insufficient amounts in the diet.

Consequences of vitamin D deficiency can be:[6]

- Weakened bones and fractures
- Higher risk of infectious disease
- Increased risk of cancer – breast, colon and prostate
- Increased risk of children developing Type I diabetes
- Exacerbation of Type II diabetes
- Muscle weakness, aches, and pains

At greatest risk are those who live at higher latitudes, where significant amounts of sunshine are limited to summer months, and those who avoid exposure to sunlight.

Moderate sunlight exposure on bare skin is the most effective source of vitamin D. Excessive exposure to the point of sunburn will not create more vitamin D and should be avoided.

Vitamin D supplementation can be effective but should always be monitored by a health care professional to avoid rare but possible toxicity from taking too much.

Here are some additional considerations:

- People with dark-skin may need more exposure to sunlight than fair-skinned people to generate the same amount of vitamin D.
- Sunlight shining through glass does not activate vitamin D formation in the skin.
- Sunscreen products impair vitamin D production from sunlight exposure.
- Food sources provide limited amounts of vitamin D. For example, you would have to drink 10 tall glasses of vitamin D fortified milk each day to get a minimal level of vitamin D.
- Some foods that have a higher vitamin D content are :

    - Sardines
    - Salmon
    - Tuna
    - Shrimp
    - Butter
    - Sunflower seeds
    - Liver
    - Eggs

- Vitamin D is crucial for calcium absorption in your digestive tract. Without sufficient vitamin D, calcium supplementation is virtually ineffective.

- Sunlight exposure will not lead to excess vitamin D as your body will only generate what it needs.
- Excessive vitamin D supplementation can lead to vitamin D toxicity.
- Symptoms of chronic vitamin D deficiency can take months of supplementation and sunlight exposure to correct.

Due to the high incidence of vitamin D deficiency and its serious consequences, it is advised that you get your vitamin D levels checked. This is done with a simple blood test called the 25-hydroxyvitamin D test, or 25(OH)D. Your doctor or health care professional can order this test and interpret the results.

If you are vitamin D deficient, supplementation with vitamin D3 is recommended as this is the form made by the skin when exposed to sunlight.

You should not supplement without first determining your body's vitamin D levels as there is a risk of vitamin D toxicity from excess supplementation.

If you are not vitamin D deficient, the safest way to maintain healthy levels is to get sunlight exposure on bare arms and legs (and torso if possible) a minimum of two to three times per week. Do not wear sunscreen and do not overexpose or sunburn your skin.

During times of the year when sunshine is less available, supplemental vitamin D may be advised. You multi-vitamin/mineral supplement may provide sufficient amounts but you should consult with your doctor or healthcare provider as individual needs can vary with age, health and dietary considerations.

> **Performance-Enhancing Drugs and Supplements**
>
> Nutrition Coaches, LLC does not support, endorse or recommend the use of any drugs or supplements that are designed to boost muscle mass, strength and endurance or to improve physical appearance.
>
> Some common examples are:
> - Creatine
> - Anabolic steroids
> - Steroid precursors – ex. androstenedione ("andro"), DHEA.
>
> **The possible long-term health dangers of such products far outweigh any short-term benefits, and the use of such products compromises the purity of sport.**

SHAKES, BARS AND GOO

Protein Powder and Shakes

There are hundreds of brands of protein powders available that offer different types of protein and many combinations of vitamins, minerals and herbs.

Proteins commonly used in these powder mixes are:

- Dairy – whey, casein
- Egg and egg white
- Pea
- Rice
- Soy

Whey, casein and egg have high biological values – a measure of how well and quickly your body uses the protein – but they are also high on the list of potential food allergens. Pea and rice proteins are low-allergenic but are less bio-available.

Soy protein powder is common and highly touted for its health benefits, but that may not be the whole story. Many health experts believe that soy can disrupt hormone balance, block absorption of some nutrients and suppress thyroid function. Until this controversy is resolved, it makes sense to err on the side of caution and minimize consumption of soy protein products.

The promotional marketing of protein powders is powerful and convincing, with pictures of six-pack abs and lean muscular bodies. Don't be fooled.

Although convenient and tasty, most protein powders are highly-processed and loaded with sugar, artificial colors, flavors, sweeteners and other less-than-healthy ingredients.

When it comes to nutrition, performance and health, protein powders are not on par with real-food proteins such as eggs, meats and fish.

If you choose to include protein powders in your diet, select a product that:

- Is whole-food based
- Has a high protein and low sugar content
- Contains no artificial sweeteners, colors and flavors
- Has fewer rather than more added supplements – you are better off getting those from real food and quality food-based supplements
- Does not use soy as its primary protein source

Whichever brand you choose, understand that protein shakes should not take the place of real food. For instance, having a protein shake for breakfast is convenient but not nearly as beneficial as having a real-food breakfast.

A further consideration is cost. On a per-serving basis, protein powders tend to be very costly, an expense that would be better used buying real-food sources such as meat and eggs.

Sport and Energy Bars

These products are designed to provide protein and carbohydrates both during and after exercise. They were originally designed as a convenient way to meet the needs of endurance athletes competing in events lasting many hours.

Many of these products are made from a mix of highly-processed carbohydrates and protein and often contain artificial flavors, colors and sweeteners.

Most sport and energy bars are little more than a candy bar in disguise.

The advantage of these products is portability and convenience. The disadvantage is their unhealthy ingredients and high cost.

When possible, choose real food first and avoid using sport and energy bars as a meal substitute, such as for breakfast. An appropriate use might be as a between-game snack, a snack while traveling or as a post-game recovery food when real food is not available.

If you use sport and energy bars, choose those that are made from real-food ingredients, have the fewest artificial ingredients, contain no artificial sweeteners, flavors and colors, are low in sugar and have a high protein content.

If you have a food allergy or intolerance, pay close attention to the ingredient list as many common food allergens (dairy, soy, nuts, etc.) can be found in these products.

Goo, Gels, and Shots

These products have become very common in recent years. For the most part, they are simply a sports drink without water, and like many commercial sports drinks, they are loaded with unhealthy ingredients. Some have stimulants, such as caffeine, added to them as well.

These products are little more than an expensive, well-marketed, flavored lump of sugar that provides no performance miracle in a packet.

If you do use them, try them in practice first to learn how your body responds and choose a brand that uses the most natural ingredients. Because they are in concentrated form, you will need to wash them down with a lot of water to avoid gastric upset, something you may not be able to do during a soccer game.

Our experience at Nutrition Coaches, LLC has shown that in most soccer situations, the use of "gels", "goo" and energy "shots" is unnecessary, impractical and often does more harm than good.

Energy Drinks

Many athletes consume energy drinks before and during competition. Most do this out of a sense of desperation, as a quick-fix to gain some imagined advantage over their competition.

This isn't a smart thing to do. If you are well-trained, well-fed and properly hydrated, you are already at your best. Drinking a can full of sugar and stimulants won't boost your performance, and may do the opposite.

Energy drinks are typically loaded with sugars, artificial sweeteners, artificial flavors and colors, caffeine and other stimulants. To rid itself of those chemicals, your body will have to use existing stores of "good" nutrients, the very ones you need to play at your best and maintain health.

Despite the advertising claims, the use of energy-drinks often leads to energy crashes and exhaustion. Other side effects may include:

- The shakes and jitters
- Extreme nervousness
- Mental mistakes from an over-hyped mind

None of these effects are desirable on a soccer field.

Don't listen to the hype. There is no magic in a can.

Top performance comes from being well-trained, well-fed, properly hydrated, and well-rested, not from being jacked-up on an energy drink. Soccer games are won by having a clear mind and playing steady and strong for the entire game.

It is the opinion of Nutrition Coaches, LLC that when it comes to consuming energy drinks, you should just say no.

SECTION IV

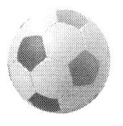

BODY FAT AND PERFORMANCE BLOCKERS

BODY FAT MANAGEMENT

Excess body fat can impair your agility, quickness and speed on the soccer field. Top players do not carry an extra ten or twenty pounds. They are well-fed, yet lean and toned. Excess body fat also dramatically increases the stress on your joints, ligaments, muscles and tendons, increasing your risk of serious injury.

Too little body fat can also impair athletic performance by limiting the amount of energy your body has available. Fatigue, low endurance and muscle weakness are common symptoms.

A chronic condition of too little body fat can cause the body to break down its own muscle mass for energy and deplete and weaken bones and connective tissues resulting in higher injury rates and more severe injuries.

How Much Should I Weigh?

Weight is an ineffective way to assess body fat. Your weight is a combined measurement of fat, bones, lean tissue and water. If your scale reveals that you have lost three pounds, you have no way of knowing if you lost fat, muscle or are just dehydrated.

A more effective way to assess your body's fat content is with a body composition measurement. This determines your fat percentage relative to your total weight. For example, a 150-pound person with 10 percent body fat would have 15 pounds of fat.

The advent of inexpensive body composition scales and devices has made the measurement of body fat percentage easy, affordable and something you can do at home.

For moderate cost, a body composition scale can be purchased at your local drug store or department store, and when properly used can measure your body fat percent with reasonable accuracy. Scales with an "Athlete" mode tend to give more accurate results for athletic bodies.

A less expensive option is a body fat caliper, which can be purchased online. You will need a second person to perform the measurement as you will not be able to measure yourself with a body fat caliper.

You should also be able to get measured at your doctor's office, training room or health club.

How Much Body Fat Do I Need?

There is no simple rule or guideline for exactly how much body fat you should carry. The percentage of body fat that is right for you will depend primarily on your gender, age, activity level and genetics.

Average body fat percentages for persons of various fitness levels are shown below.

AVERAGE BODY FAT PERCENTAGE

	Men	Women*
Non-Athlete	18 – 25%	25 – 30%
Recreational Athlete	14 – 17%	21 – 24%
Well-Trained Athlete	6 – 13%	14 – 20%

*It is normal for women to have a higher body fat percentage than men.

The measurement of body fat is not an exact science. Practically speaking, measurements of body fat can often be three points higher or lower than your actual body fat.

Therefore, it is best not to focus on the actual number but instead use multiple measurements to track relative changes in body fat over time.

In addition, two healthy people of equal fitness can have very different fat percentage numbers. This is often due to genetics.

When assessing body fat, keep in mind that you know your body better than anyone else, and you know how you feel when you play soccer.

If your body fat is a little high for your activity level but you feel quick and fit, then there is little need to be concerned. However, if you feel heavy and slow and your numbers are high, you might want to consider tuning your body to a leaner state and see how that works for you.

On the other hand, if your numbers are consistently low and you feel fatigued and weak, it might be time to improve your dietary intake and put on a few pounds to restore your energy level.

CAUTION!	Extremely high or low body fat percent numbers can often indicate a dangerous health condition that is best handled with the help of a healthcare professional.

Both situations require common sense and paying attention to how you feel. Remember, your goal as a soccer player is to eat healthy meals that fuel your body for top performance and maintain healthy body fat levels.

Body Fat Reduction

Here are some basic guidelines for reducing body fat:

- Losing significant amounts of excess body fat is best done during the off season.
- Set a realistic goal of losing 1 to 2 pounds of fat per week and seek support from a friend, family member or significant other. It is often difficult to do alone.

- Focus on eating whole foods from your Diet Plan and carefully monitor your portions of protein, fat and carbohydrates.
- Reduce or eliminate consumption of all processed grain products such as breads, cereals, pastas and crackers. Limiting consumption of whole grain products can also help.
- Eat three meals per day and do not skip breakfast.
- Space your meals five to six hours apart.
- Avoid snacking but if you must snack choose a small, protein-based snack. Strong hunger or cravings between meals indicates improper type of food or portions at the last meal.
- Strong food cravings can often be eased or eliminated with a short bit of intense exercise such as walking up and down stairs multiple times or a brisk walk.
- Finish dinner at least three hours before bedtime and get a full night's sleep. Sleep deprivation can alter metabolism and that can lead to weight retention or gain.
- Do not eat after dinner and, if possible, allow 11 to 12 hours between dinner and breakfast. This will encourage your body to burn fat while you sleep.
- Eat slowly and stick with modest portions. Finish your meals when slightly less than full. The "I'm full" signal will catch up in 10 to 20 minutes.
- Exercise is crucial to "burning" body fat.
- Build your exercise program until you can work out four to six times each week for 30 to 60 minutes per session. The goal is to get your heart rate (beats per minute) into your target range.

Target Heart Rate

There are several methods to calculate your target heart rate. A mathematical formula called The Karvonen Formula works well and takes age into account but you will need to know your resting pulse rate.[1]

A Karvonen Formula heart-rate calculator is easily found with an online search.

Here is a simpler rule to follow if you don't want to measure your pulse rate:

- If you are too out of breath to maintain a conversation, slow down
- If you can talk easily or sing a song, pick up the intensity

- Your exercise can be steady or take the form of intervals. An example of steady exercise is a long run or bike ride at a constant speed.

- Interval training involves short periods of higher intensity exercise followed by less intense activity or rest:

  o Perform a specific exercise at high intensity for a set period of time (usually 15 seconds to two minutes) then slow down or rest before repeating the sequence.

  o Your rest time should be about two to four times as long as your interval time.

  o Interval training should be gradually brought into your exercise routine due to its intense nature.

- Whatever activity you choose – bike, run, hike, swim, play sports – for your workout, be sure to add some variety to keep it enjoyable. And to build and maintain strong bones, some load-bearing exercise, such as weight lifting, should be part of your weekly routine. An effective way to burn fat and tone muscles is to lift weights on alternate days from interval training.

| **CAUTION!** | Always consult with your healthcare provider before beginning any new exercise program. |

Ideally, allow three hours after eating before exercising. This will encourage your body to access its own fat instead of burning what you just ate.

If you break the dietary rules, for example by eating a piece of pie before bedtime or snacking on sweets between meals, you can knock your body out of fat-burning mode for many hours or even a full day.

During that time, your progress can stop or even reverse. That is where your resolve and your partner's support come into play. Once you achieve your desired weight / body fat percentage, then you can occasionally break the pattern, but not until then.

Food Sensitivity

Your health and soccer performance can be negatively affected if you suffer from an allergic reaction or intolerance to a food or foods.

Conditions commonly associated with food sensitivities are:

- Chronic or frequent infections
- Canker sores
- Chronic diarrhea or constipation
- Irritable bowel syndrome
- Insomnia
- Anxiety, hyperactivity, irritability

- Inability to concentrate
- Joint pain, back pain
- Asthma, nasal/airway congestion
- Acne, eczema, rashes
- Edema (swelling)
- Fatigue
- Headaches, migraines
- Sinus problems
- Seizures
- Celiac disease

Food allergies and other adverse reactions to food are reported to occur in 25 percent of young children. The cause is believed to be excessive regular consumption of a limited number of foods (that are often hidden in industrial foods), and high levels of preservatives and artificial colors and flavors.[2] Food and environmental contaminants such as pesticide residues, air pollution and impaired digestion can also play a role.

Statistics also reveal that during the past decade, the incidence of food allergies has dramatically increased.[3]

Food Allergy

An allergic reaction to food is an immune system response to food molecules that are absorbed into the blood stream during digestion.

Resulting symptoms can develop in minutes to 24 hours after food consumption and can range from barely discernible to, in extreme cases, death from airway constriction or anaphylactic shock.

According to the U.S. Food and Drug Administration (www.fda.gov) products made from the following foods account for 90 percent of food allergic reactions:

- Milk
- Eggs
- Shellfish
- Fish
- Tree nuts
- Peanuts
- Wheat
- Soy

In addition, some people can experience exercise-induced food allergies or, if sensitive to airborne allergens, can experience a food allergy from eating fresh fruits and vegetables that have proteins similar to those found in airborne allergens such as pollen.

A food allergy can also be "developed" by eating the same food too frequently and not having enough of a varied diet. An example would be eating eggs for breakfast every morning for an extended period. This is not guaranteed to cause an allergy to eggs, but it can increase the probability.

Due to the many ingredients used in industrial foods, those foods may contain a variety of potential food allergens. For example, a commercially produced cookie may contain milk, eggs, wheat, soy and tree nuts – five common food allergens.

In addition, if "natural flavors" is listed as an ingredient, you have no way of knowing if food allergens are in that food because by law, a natural flavor can contain almost any substance extracted, distilled or otherwise derived from plant or animal matter. Some companies identify common allergens in their products but many do not.

The key points to take from this discussion are:

- Real, whole foods have only one ingredient so you know what you are eating.
- Eating a food you are allergic to day after day can "wear out" your immune system.

- If you eat a varied, real-food diet you are less likely to "develop" a food allergy.
- A food allergy can negatively affect your health and soccer performance.

Food Intolerance

Negative reactions to foods that do not involve an immune system response are commonly called "intolerances".

Common food intolerance symptoms include:

- Bloating
- Congestion and coughing
- Constipation
- Diarrhea
- Fatigue
- Flatulence
- Gastric discomfort
- Headaches
- Hives
- Nausea
- Rapid pulse rate
- Weight gain (or hard to lose)

These reactions may be in response to chemicals in foods such as monosodium glutamate (MSG), pesticides, colorings, flavorings, sweeteners and preservatives, or they may be caused by an inability to digest a particular food.

Foods that commonly cause intolerance are:

- Dairy (cow's milk)
- Wheat
- Fructose
- Yeast

Dairy products have a very high rate of intolerance. You may find that surprising as they are heavily promoted as being healthy and, in the United States, are consumed at the rate of nearly 600 pounds per person per year, primarily in the form of milk, cheese and yogurt.

Depending on your genetics, your chances of having a dairy intolerance may be quite high. Following are statistical estimates from the National Institute of Health (www.hih.gov) on dairy intolerance rates of peoples from various ethnic backgrounds:

RATE OF INTOLERANCE TO DAIRY PRODUCTS

Ethnicity	Rate of Intolerance
Asians	95%
African Americans	60 – 80%
Hispanics	50 – 80%
Mediterranean Peoples	70%
Native American Indians	80 – 100%
Caucasians	20%
Northern Europeans	Less than 10%
Other World Population	75%

The reason for high rates of dairy intolerance is that the digestive enzyme (lactase) that breaks down milk sugar (lactose) is highest in infants – to digest breast milk – but diminishes during childhood and adolescence to only 5 to 10 percent of infant levels.

Only about 25 percent of people worldwide, mostly of northern European descent, retain enough lactase to digest and absorb dairy products efficiently throughout adult life.

Checking for a Food Sensitivity

A complete discussion on food sensitivity testing is beyond the scope of this book but the following three techniques can be effective:

<u>Blood test</u>

Modern blood tests can accurately determine food and non-food sensitivities. Consult with your healthcare provider to determine which tests are available to you. These tests can be expensive and may or may not be covered by health insurance, so know your upfront costs before testing.

CAUTION!	Do not use the Elimination Food Allergy Test or the Allergy Pulse Test method if you tend toward strong allergic reactions. Severe allergic reactions, such as airway constriction, can be life threatening.

Elimination Food Allergy Test

This method involves eliminating all potential allergenic foods from your diet for a period of at least one week and then re-introducing single foods every two days and monitoring your body's response.

Allergy Pulse Test

This method involves sitting quietly and measuring your heart rate both before and one minute after putting a small quantity of the food in question under your tongue. An increase or decrease in heart rate of 4 to 6 beats per minute or more can indicate a reaction to that food.

A blood test is the preferred method because of its accuracy and convenience. The other two methods can be done on your own, the Allergy Pulse Test being quicker and easier but less reliable than the Elimination Diet method. More information on both of these methods is readily available online.

Sometimes it can be as easy as eliminating a suspected problem food from your diet and then monitoring how you feel for the next few days to a week. If you feel significantly better, you may be having a sensitivity issue with that particular food.

If you have intolerance to a particular food, you should significantly reduce or eliminate consumption of that food.

If you are allergic to a food, complete avoidance is usually necessary. This can be challenging as a food can appear in many forms.

For example, to avoid dairy products, you will need to stay away from all foods that contain milk, butter, cheese, yogurt, buttermilk, cottage cheese, casein, powdered milk and whey.

Since dairy products can be found in many foods, such as breads, desserts and even some luncheon meats, you will need to read food labels. You will also need to ask about food ingredients when eating in restaurants – the staff in most restaurants will be happy to make adjustments as needed.

If you eliminate a food from your diet, be sure to eat appropriate amounts of other foods that supply similar nutrients as the food you eliminated.

Digestive Tract Health

Your digestive tract is a nearly 30-foot-long tube that breaks down and absorbs what you eat and drink. If your digestive tract is not healthy and working efficiently, your ability to absorb energy and nutrition from your food will be impaired. As a consequence, your soccer performance can suffer and so can your health.

Some common conditions often associated with an impaired digestive system:

- Constipation/diarrhea
- Bloating/gas
- Allergies
- Headaches
- Chronic inflammation
- Indigestion/heartburn/acid reflux
- Irritable bowel syndrome
- Yeast/fungal infections
- Skin disruptions

Given the seriousness of these conditions, it makes sense to keep your digestive tract healthy and working efficiently.

How Your Digestive Tract Works

Digestion begins in the mouth. Chewing breaks down food into smaller pieces and mixes it with saliva. The more thoroughly food is chewed, the easier time the rest of the digestive tract will have processing it.

After food is swallowed, it is mixed with acid and enzymes in the stomach. The acid is about as strong as lemon juice, and its primary functions are to begin digestion of the protein molecules and to kill microbes that may have been swallowed with the food. You stomach acid is a primary part of your immune system.

> **Did You Know?**
> The absorptive area of the small intestine has approximately the same surface area as a tennis court.

Once the food is thoroughly mixed in the stomach, it passes into the small intestine where it is further broken down by digestive juices and absorbed by various means into the blood stream.

What remains is passed into the large intestine where some additional fluids and minerals are absorbed, and some of the fiber from the food is further digested by bacteria that live there. The byproducts of digestion are then excreted.

Digestive tract problems

The process of digestion is complex and interactive. For instance, living in your large intestine are many different kinds of "friendly" bacteria, which are often referred to as "gut flora."

It is estimated that there are 100 trillion bacteria cells in a healthy digestive tract, which is about 10 times the number of cells in the rest of your body. But contrary to what most people think about bacteria, these are not bad bacteria. Instead, they are beneficial and very important to your health.

Here are a few of the things those good bacteria do for you:

- Produce enzymes that help you digest plant and vegetable matter

- Stimulate your immune system
- Help maintain balanced body chemistry
- Produce some B vitamins and vitamin K (critical to blood clotting)
- Keep unfriendly bacteria and microbes from gaining a foothold

Clearly, maintaining the health of your intestinal bacteria is in your best interest. However, sometimes the bacteria colony can get damaged by diet or medications.

For instance, when you take an oral antibiotic, it kills the bad bacteria that are making you sick but it can also kill much of your friendly gut flora. When that happens, a form of yeast called Candida can flourish and take its place, often causing significant health problems such as:

- Bloating and digestive tract pain
- Skin problems (acne)
- Fatigue and trouble concentrating
- Anxiety and mood swings
- Headaches
- Strong cravings for sweets and breads

Another digestive problem that is becoming more common is chronic low stomach acid (Hypochlorhydria).[4] This condition can lead to a host of problems such as:

- Malabsorption of proteins
- Poor mineral absorption
- Higher risk of stomach infections
- Vitamin B12 deficiency
- Gas/bloating/Irritable Bowel Syndrome

- Heartburn, acid reflux, GERD
- Anemia
- Candida overgrowth

One study showed that out of 200 asthmatic children, 80 percent had low stomach acid levels.[5]

There are many factors that can disrupt normal digestive health – improper diet, medications, alcohol consumption, infection and illness are a few. It is beyond the scope of this book to offer remedies to digestive tract issues, but if you have digestive problems or are experiencing some of the conditions listed above, you should consult your healthcare provider and begin working on a fix.

It may be as simple as supplementing with probiotics (friendly gut flora in a capsule) for a few weeks or months, or it may require some digestive enzyme support or even stomach acid supplementation.

Whatever the fix, get it done because digestive problems can easily lead to far more severe and chronic health problems down the road, none of which will benefit your soccer performance.

You can eat great food and take quality supplements, but if your digestive system is not properly breaking down and absorbing its contents, you won't be getting the nutrients and energy needed to play at the top of your game.

SECTION V

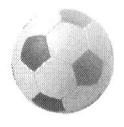

DIETARY FAT DEMYSTIFIED

This section is somewhat more technical than the previous sections due to the innate complexity of the topic. To fully explore dietary fat is a book in itself. Presented here is an overview that will leave you with a basic working-knowledge of the often confusing topic of dietary fat.

The public health message about dietary fat during the last half century is that fat is bad, saturated fat is really bad and that if you eat fat, you get fat.

Billions of dollars are spent each year on low-fat foods and pills that block absorption of fat from the digestive system, and even though fat consumption has declined during the last 40 years, obesity and heart disease are occurring at rates never before seen in history.

When you consider that mankind has been eating fat for many thousands of years and has only recently become so chronically ill, a logical conclusion might be that it is time to change the public message.

But that is easier said than done because the role of dietary fat in the human body is a very complex and controversial subject, even among experts in the field.

It is beyond the scope of this book to engage in a detailed discussion on dietary fats. Instead, here's a simple and practical approach:

- Not all fats are the same
- There are good, health-promoting fats

- There are bad, unhealthy fats
- Moderate amounts of good fats are a necessary part of your diet
- Bad fats should be avoided
- Eating fat doesn't necessarily make you fat
- Humans have eaten fat for many thousands of years

The Role of Fat in the Body

Fat has many important functions:

- Providing energy for extended exercise or to combat hunger
- Transporting fat soluble vitamins (vitamins A, D, E and K)
- Assisting in hormone production and function
- Insulating the body against temperature extremes
- Cushioning bones and vital organs against shock
- Assisting the body in efficient use of carbohydrates and protein
- Maintaining healthy skin (fat is a primary component of all cell membranes)

In addition, dietary fat is essential for proper fetal development during pregnancy, milk production in nursing mothers and normal development of the child.

There are entire cultures that eat large amounts of dietary fat and are very healthy. Other groups survive well on lower fat diets. How much healthy fat you need in your diet for optimum energy production can depend largely on your genetics.

What is Fat?

In simple terms, fats are chains of carbon atoms with attached hydrogen atoms. The more hydrogen atoms that are attached, the more saturated the fat.

In general, the more saturated the fat, the more stable it is when exposed to heat (cooking), light and oxygen. In other words, it is less likely to become rancid as easily as unsaturated fat.

Fats are classified as fatty acids. The length of the carbon chain identifies them as being:

- Long chain fatty acids (12 to 24 carbon atoms)
    - Found in meat, fish, seeds, vegetable oils
- Medium chain fatty acids (6 to 10 carbon atoms)
    - Found in coconut and palm oils
- Short chain fatty acids (less than 6 carbon atoms)
    - Found in dairy butterfat

The length of the carbon chain affects how the body processes the fat. Most long chain fatty acids are absorbed in the digestive tract and transported through the lymphatic system before entering the blood stream near the heart.

Medium and short chain fatty acids normally bypass the lymphatic system and enter the bloodstream directly and more rapidly.

Hence, long chain fats, such as animal fat, provide a long-lasting, steady source of energy while shorter chain fats tend to be more quickly processed and used.

That is why eating a meal that is high in animal fat right before a game is not a good idea. Conversely, that is also why fat can make a meal satisfying; it digests slowly and provides slow, steady energy after the meal.

Fats rarely exist as single fatty acids but instead form triglycerides, which are three fatty acids attached to a glycerol molecule. This is the form in which most fat exists in the body and in food.

Calories from carbohydrates, protein and fat that are ingested during a meal and are not immediately used by tissues are converted into triglycerides and transported to fat cells to be stored.

When the body needs energy and none is available from digestion, hormones trigger the release of triglycerides from body fat to provide that energy.

Triglyceride levels measured in blood tests are simply a measure of how much fat is circulating in your blood.

> **Fat Facts**
> - "Fat" and "oil" are both forms of dietary fat. The difference is that fat is a solid at room temperature and oil is a liquid.
> - Fat provides 9 calories (kcal) of energy per gram
> - Protein and Carbohydrates provide 4 calories (kcal) per gram
> - One pound of body fat contains 3,500 calories (kcal)
> - Fat provides most of the energy during a long distance run.
>
> **A 150-pound person running an Olympic marathon (26.2 miles) will burn about the same amount of energy that is contained in just one pound of body fat!**

Types of Fat

There are three types of dietary fat:

Saturated Fats

- Tend to be solid or mostly solid at room temperature and below
- Are less likely to go rancid and form health-damaging compounds at cooking temperatures and or when exposed to oxygen or light
- Natural sources:
  - Animal fats
  - Tropical oils such as coconut and palm oil

Monounsaturated Fats

- Tend to be liquid at room temperature and solid when refrigerated
- Are relatively stable and less likely to become rancid at cooking temperatures or when exposed to oxygen or light
- When needed, these fats can be made in the body from saturated fats
- Natural sources:
    - Olive and sesame oil
    - Avocados
    - Almonds, cashews, pecans, and peanuts

Polyunsaturated Fats

- Tend to be liquid at room temperature and when refrigerated
- Are "essential" because the body cannot make them and therefore they must be obtained from food
- Two common types are:
    - Linoleic acid (omega-6)
    - Linolenic acid (omega-3)
- Tend to be unstable and easily form health-damaging compounds when heated and/or exposed to light and oxygen such as during cooking or during processing and extraction
- Should be kept refrigerated and protected from light and oxygen

Natural, Healthy Fats

- Linoleic (omega-6): nuts, seeds, beans and their oils
- Linolenic (omega-3): flaxseed, fish (salmon, sardines), walnuts and chia seeds

When eaten in moderation and in their natural form, all of these natural fats are healthy. The best way to get maximum nutritional benefit from nuts, seeds and beans is to simply eat them in their raw, natural form.

Cold pressed oils from nuts, seeds and beans will retain many of the original nutrients, but as you will see below, that is not the type of oil that is commonly available in stores.

Unnatural, Industrial Fats

Apart from olive oil, most oils available in grocery stores are refined oils from grains, seeds and beans. They are mostly colorless, sold in clear bottles and have little taste.

Examples are:

- Canola oil
- Corn oil
- Cottonseed oil
- Safflower oil
- Soybean oil
- Sunflower oil
- Vegetable oil

The manufacturing process that creates these refined oils often involves solvent-chemical extraction, bleaching, and high-temperature deodorization. The result is a finished product that has been stripped of its nutritional value by the manufacturing process but has a long shelf life.

Some of the oils are also hydrogenated or partially hydrogenated – a process that adds hydrogen to the fat molecule and turns normally liquid oils into a butter-like consistency that is less likely to go rancid.

Margarine, a common butter substitute, is an example of hydrogenated oil, usually made from corn or soy.

The disadvantage of hydrogenation is that it creates trans fatty acids (trans fats) – substances being strongly linked to numerous serious health problems[1,2,3,4,5,6] such as:

- Diabetes
- Heart disease
- Obesity
- Systemic inflammation
- Breast cancer

The following are some industrial foods that often contain trans-fats:

- Fried foods – doughnuts, French fries, chicken nuggets, and hard taco shells, chips, etc.
- Commercial baked goods such as cookies, crackers, cakes, muffins, pie crusts, pizza dough, and some breads
- Margarines and vegetable shortenings
- Pre-mixed cake and pancake mixes, and chocolate drink mixes
- Snack foods such as potato chips, candies and microwave popcorn
- Some frozen dinners

This is another case where industrialization of food has made it unhealthy.

It may or may not be a coincidence that the rapid rise in heart disease in the last century coincides with the introduction and increased use of hydrogenated and refined oils in the food supply.

Based on the evidence now emerging and the fact that industrial foods rarely outdo their natural counterparts when it comes to health, it is the opinion of Nutrition Coaches, LLC that consumption of refined oils, hydrogenated and partially hydrogenated oils, and the resulting trans fats are best avoided.

Cholesterol

There is probably no nutritional substance surrounded by more controversy, confusion and fear than cholesterol. To stay within the intent of this book, only a brief discussion of the subject and some very basic recommendations are provided. Further research by you into the health effects of cholesterol is highly recommended.

Cholesterol is a waxy substance made up of fat and protein that is found in animal products such as animal fat, eggs, etc. Cholesterol does not exist in plant products.

Your liver produces about 80 percent of the cholesterol in your body with the rest coming from dietary sources. How much it makes depends on how much cholesterol you consume and your body's requirements.

In humans, cholesterol serves three essential functions:

- It is a key component of cell membranes and structures and as such is a building block for body tissues.
- It is used by glands to manufacture hormones (the chemical messengers of the body) such as estrogen and testosterone.
- It is used by the liver to produce bile, which breaks down fat in the digestive system.

How much cholesterol you should get from your diet is a very controversial subject, as high cholesterol levels in the blood are in some ways tied to coronary heart disease, a leading cause of death in modern-food societies.

However, there is much controversy in the medical and scientific community surrounding the true connection between heart disease and high cholesterol.

Some researchers argue that high cholesterol in the body is a strong indicator and causative factor of heart disease. Others argue that there is no statistical difference in mortality rates between people with high and low cholesterol and, therefore, cholesterol is not a significant factor.

Consumption of saturated fat, which may alter cholesterol levels, is touted as health-damaging by some, while others believe that saturated fat in its natural form is health-promoting and not a factor in heart disease. Certainly, hydrogenated oils and trans fats are not healthy in anyone's thinking.

When you add factors such as refined carbohydrate consumption, physical activity and lifestyle habits, the complexity of the situation is greatly compounded.[7]

There is validity to both sides of the argument about fat and heart disease. But it is important to note that some cultures consume vastly different amounts of saturated fat and cholesterol and yet remain relatively free from heart disease. This reality points to genetics being a powerful factor in this issue, but certainly not the only factor.

Complicating the subject more is the relentless promotion of the negative effects of high cholesterol by the multi-billion dollar industry that has grown around cholesterol-lowering drugs and low-cholesterol foods. There is much profit in selling pills, and that can influence the mindset of many people, scientific or not.

Clearly there are many overlapping factors that play a role in any medical health issue, and that can make it unwise to simply focus on one, such as cholesterol, as being the sole culprit in heart disease.

Many gaps remain in understanding how diet, cholesterol and heart disease are interrelated. Therefore, until more is known, a reasonable approach is to maintain healthy lifestyle habits, exercise regularly, eat real, whole foods and limit consumption of industrial foods.

In general, people who follow those simple guidelines tend to have "healthy" cholesterol levels. However, there are always exceptions, so if you have any concerns or if you haven't already done so, get your cholesterol levels checked with a simple blood test.

If your results indicate a problem, talk with your health care provider and politely ask him or her to back up any recommendations with documentation. Why?

Because the advertising influence of drug companies can extend into a doctor's office just as easily as into your home, and if your doctor's only recent information is that provided by those who profit from the sale of cholesterol-lowering medications, then you may not be getting the entire story.

And always do your own research so that you will be well informed before making any major dietary or medical decisions. An Internet search for "The Cholesterol Myth" can reveal some very interesting counterpoint information.

The Essential Fats

Omega-3 and omega-6 fatty acids are polyunsaturated fats that are classified as "essential" because the human body must have them to be healthy and can only get them from dietary sources.

These two fatty acids play a vital role in virtually every biological function in the human body such as regulation of blood-clotting, blood pressure, heart rate, inflammation and immune response.[8]

Did You Know?
There are three types of Omega-3 fats. They are:
- ALA (alpha-linolenic acid)
- EPA (eicosapentaenoic acid)
- DHA (docosahexaneonic acid)

Essential fats also play a powerful role in mental wellness, injury healing, recovery from exercise, burning body fat and cellular energy production.[8] Maintaining a healthy intake of essential fats is vital to health and top soccer performance.

But you can't just consume a lot of both of these fatty acids and expect beneficial results. It is both the amount and ratio of omega-6 to omega-3 that needs to be correct for optimum health and performance.

It is estimated that ancient man eating a diet of green plants, fruits, nuts, berries, fish and meats consumed nearly equal amounts of both omega-6 and omega-3 fatty acids, a ratio of 1:1.[9]

With the introduction of modern, industrial foods such as grain products, grain-fed livestock, farmed-fish, dairy products and processed vegetable oils, the ratio of omega-6 to omega-3 in the United States' diet has increased to between 10:1 and 25:1, and perhaps much higher.[10]

Since human genes have changed little since ancient times, it makes sense to steer away from industrial foods that unbalance the essential fat ratio and consume foods that are more balanced.

A ratio of 1:1 to 4:1 is generally considered optimal, although figuring out exactly how much of each you consume is not easy. One internationally recognized expert recommends the following:[8]

OMEGA-6 AND OMEGA-3 DAILY RECOMMENDATIONS

	Daily Requirement (grams/day)	Estimated Optimum* (grams/day)
Omega-6	3	9
Omega-3	2	6

*Individual needs may vary based on body size, state of health, stress, activity level, season, and climate.

A simple and effective approach to balance your essential fat intake is to add a variety of omega-3 sources to your whole-food diet.

CAUTION! Excessive consumption of either omega-6 or omega-3 can unbalance body chemistry and lead to health problems. Stay within the above daily consumption guidelines. More is not better.

ESSENTIAL FAT CONTENT OF COMMON FOODS & OILS*

Source	Omega-6	Omega-3	Omega-6 to Omega-3 Ratio
	Grams Per Tablespoon		
Flaxseed Oil	1.7	7.2	1 : 4
Flaxseed, whole	0.6	2.3	1 : 4
Flaxseed, ground	0.4	1.6	1 : 4
Chia Seeds, dry	0.6	1.8	1 : 4
Chia Seeds, gel (8:1)	---	0.2	1 : 4
Fish Oil	0.3	3.8	1 : 13
Butter, whole fat	0.4	---	9 : 1
Coconut Oil, virgin	0.2	---	>100 : 1
Olive Oil, virgin	1.3	0.1	12 : 1
	Grams Per ¼ cup (about a handful)		
Almonds	2.9	---	>100 : 1
Peanuts	5.7	---	>100 : 1
Pecans	5.6	0.3	21 : 1
Pumpkin Seeds	7.1	0.1	71 : 1
Sunflower Seeds	2.6	---	---
Walnuts, black	10.3	0.6	16 : 1
Oatmeal, plain dry	0.4	---	22 : 1
Wheat Germ	1.5	0.2	7 : 1
Avocado, pureed	1.0	---	15 : 1
	Grams Per Ounce		
Salmon, Coho	---	0.3	1 : 20
Sardines	1.0	0.4	2 : 1
Trout, cooked	0.1	0.4	6 : 1
Beef, grain fed[11]	variable		8 : 1
Beef, pastured[11]	variable		2 : 1
Egg, standard	variable		15 : 1
Egg, pastured[12, 13]	variable		2 : 1

*Source: USDA National Nutrient Database for Standard Reference, Release 23 (2010)
--- indicates less than 0.1 grams

Flaxseeds, flaxseed oil, chia seeds, salmon, trout and fish oil are high in omega-3 fatty acids but relatively low in omega-6. Nuts, seeds and grain products tend to be the opposite.

To balance your essential fat intake, choose various food sources. For example, a handful of almonds and a tablespoon of flaxseeds will provide the recommended daily requirement of three grams of omega-6 and two grams of omega-3.

In place of flaxseed, you could eat six ounces of salmon. Food sources of omega-3 are preferred. Flax oil and fish oil supplements are best used therapeutically.

Be sure to take fish oil with meals and only use brands that have been tested to be contaminate-free. Keep fish oil supplements refrigerated.

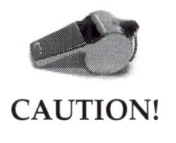

CAUTION!	Before supplementing your diet with flaxseed oil, fish oil or other concentrated source of omega-3 fatty acids, you should consult with your health care provider to avoid any potential side effects and interactions with medications.

Flaxseed

Flaxseed must be ground to be digestible. Ground seeds provide vitamins, trace minerals and lignans. Flaxseed oil is a concentrated source of omega-3 fatty acids but contains few of these other nutrients.

Both ground flaxseed and flaxseed oil should be refrigerated as exposure to air, light and heat cause rapid spoilage. Whole flaxseed is more durable but is best handled in a similar way.

Did You Know?
Lignans are plant-based compounds with anti-bacterial, anti-viral, anti-fungal and anti-cancer properties.

Maximum nutritional benefit is obtained by grinding individual servings of whole flaxseeds in a small grinder, such as a coffee grinder, and consuming soon thereafter. Drink plenty of fluid as ground flaxseeds absorb five times their volume in liquid.

Commercial ground flaxseed (flax meal) is convenient but depending on processing, packaging and shelf-time, it may be partially rancid by the time you buy it. The same can apply to flaxseed oil.

Rancid flaxseed oil smells like paint and stale flax meal tastes bitter and has a strong smell. Both should be discarded.

Whole flaxseed and flaxseed oil is commonly available in most natural food stores and online.

Chia Seeds

These high protein seeds are an excellent source of essential fats. They are gaining popularity as an endurance running food because their carbohydrate content is slowly absorbed by the body due to the high soluble-fiber content of the seeds.

The essential fat, protein and carbohydrate content of chia seeds make them suitable for use in a pre-game meal or post-game recovery food or drink.

The best way to use chia seeds is to mix the dry seeds with water to form a chia gel. The seeds absorb up to nine times their own volume in water as seen in the following photographs.

To make chia gel, mix 1 part dry seeds with 6 to 9 parts water in a sealable container. Use less water to make a thicker gel. Stir or shake the mixture immediately and again after a minute to prevent clumping. The seeds will fully gel in 10 to 15 minutes and stay fresh for up to two weeks when refrigerated.

Chia gel can be mixed with smoothies and protein shakes, oatmeal, sauces, rice, stir fries, salads and vegetables. The gel is mostly flavorless, easily digested and adds a smooth texture to foods.

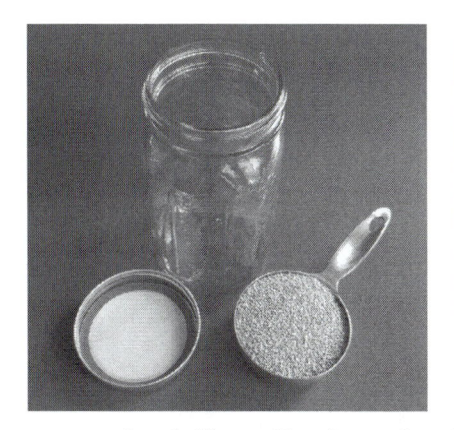

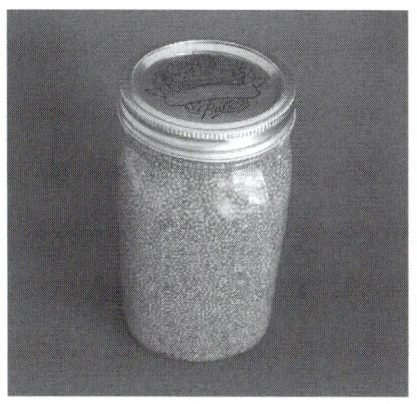

One-half cup of dry chia seeds and water makes a quart of chia gel.

A common amount of chia gel to consume is one to three tablespoons, one to three times daily. This will provide a healthy supply of dietary fiber and essential fat. If you consume chia seeds dry, be sure to drink plenty of water with them.

Chia seeds are available online and in some natural food stores.

Recommendations for Dietary Fat

Dietary fat, both saturated and unsaturated, has been a natural part of the human diet for thousands of years. In its natural form and when consumed in moderation, dietary fat is a good source of energy and has many health benefits.

Highly-refined oils and hydrogenated and trans-fats are not a healthy choice. Unfortunately, they are commonly used in restaurants so be wary of ordering fatty foods when dining out. They can also be found in many industrial foods, particularly in deep-fried foods and commercial baked goods.

Fat is energy-dense, so use moderation when consuming it. A reasonable starting point is a fat intake of 15 to 20 percent of total daily caloric intake with one third of that being essential fat.[8]

This amount of fat is common in traditional diets that support health without degenerative diseases. However, depending on your genetics and the demands you put on your body, your fat intake needs may vary considerably.

Fat does not necessarily make you fat. Any excess calories from carbohydrates, protein, or fat will be turned into body fat. Your body accepts all forms of food energy and will either use it or store it. It is indiscriminate when it comes to energy.

A general rule for eating nuts and seeds is a small handful or two per day. They are nutrient-rich and have high fat content so smaller quantities are sufficient.

> **What is Virgin Oil?**
>
> Virgin oils are obtained solely by mechanical means that do not alter the oil in any way. They have not undergone any treatment other than washing, decanting, centrifuging, and filtering.
>
> Extra virgin oil is the highest quality of virgin oil.

Extra-virgin or virgin olive oil is a good choice for use on salads or for light stir-frying of foods. Flax oil is also good on salads but should not be used for cooking as it easily degrades with heat.

Virgin coconut oil is flavorful and can be used much like butter – as a condiment on steamed vegetables, for cooking, on whole-grain toast, etc. Coconut is not a source of essential fats.

When cooking, lower temperatures are better as heat degrades fats and oils. Oil heated to its smoking point should be discarded. Smoking point temperatures of various oils and fats are easily found with an online search.

If you have any concerns about or have a health condition that requires restriction of fat intake in any way, be sure to follow the advice of your health care provider.

<u>Healthy Fats</u>

- Olive oil
    - o Choose cold pressed, extra virgin
    - o Suitable for cooking and as a condiment

- o Store in cool dark place
- o Will become cloudy or solidify if refrigerated but will return to normal when warmed
- Coconut
  - o Choose cold pressed, virgin coconut oil
  - o Forms: oil, milk, raw flakes
  - o Has a high level of medium chain fatty acids that provide immediate energy and are less likely to be stored as body fat
  - o Contains lauric acid, which has immune-boosting and anti-microbial properties
  - o Virgin coconut oil can be used like butter – as a condiment and for cooking
  - o Flavor can vary by brand
  - o Can be stored at room temperature (melts at 76 °F)
- Butter
  - o Choose raw, organic
  - o Can be used for cooking and as a condiment
  - o Pasteurization degrades its health benefits
  - o Must be refrigerated
- Fish
  - o High fat fish – wild salmon, sardines, mackerel, herring, lake trout, etc. are good sources of omega-3 fatty acids
  - o Know your source to avoid contaminants in fish and shellfish (mercury for example)

- Avocado (guacamole)
    - High in nutrients, fiber and monounsaturated fats
    - Adds a unique flavor and texture to sandwiches, salads, etc.
- Eggs
    - Pastured hens lay higher omega-3 eggs
    - Organic omega-3 eggs are next best choice to eggs from pastured hens
    - Are high in antioxidants and other nutrients
- Nuts and nut oils (almonds, cashews, macadamias, pecans, peanuts, walnuts, etc.)
    - Choose organic whenever possible
    - Are a great source of healthy fats and other nutrients
    - Choose raw or lightly roasted, unsalted or lightly salted, and avoid those cooked in oil
    - Can add unique flavors to foods
    - Store all nuts and nut oils in refrigerator
- Seeds (sunflower, pumpkin, sesame, flax, chia)
    - Excellent source of healthy fats
    - Flax and chia have high omega-3 content
    - Pumpkin seeds have many health-promoting nutrients
    - Choose raw or lightly roasted, unsalted or lightly salted, and avoid those cooked in oil
    - Store all seeds and seed oils in refrigerator
    - Flax oil should not be used for cooking

- Dark Chocolate (70 percent cocoa or higher)
    - Choose less-sweet kinds
    - Contains anti-oxidants
- Animal Fat
    - Pasture-raised animals and birds eating natural food have a more balanced ratio of omega-6 to omega-3 fatty acids than grain fed animals and birds.

Unhealthy Fats

Minimize or avoid consumption of the following oils and fats:

- Refined oils:
    - Corn oil
    - Canola oil
    - Cottonseed oil
    - Safflower oil
    - Sunflower oil
    - Soybean oil
    - Vegetable oil
- Hydrogenated and partially hydrogenated oils and trans fats

Summary

Don't fear fat. In its natural form and when consumed in moderation, it is necessary and beneficial to your health.

The majority of unhealthy fats are found in industrial foods. Highly-refined and hydrogenated oils are often used in restaurants and fast food establishments.

The more you know the source of your food and the more natural your diet, the easier it is to avoid eating unhealthy dietary fats.

Balance the intake of essential fats in your diet by consuming various food sources.

SECTION VI

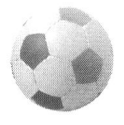

MAKE SMART FOOD CHOICES

This section provides information to help you make informed decisions about food – how to select, store, prepare and maintain nutrient quality.

Also discussed is food contamination and its potential health effects. This information is included so you can make better food choices, not to dissuade you from eating healthy foods.

For example, most people do not eat enough fruits and vegetables. To avoid those foods for contamination reasons and instead eat less-healthy foods, such as sugar-laden industrial foods, is wrong.

It is far better to eat healthy foods that may have minor contamination issues than to eat unhealthy industrial foods that are probably equally or more contaminated.

Chances are you will not be able to eat the best quality foods every meal of every day. However, being informed about food will allow you to do the best you can within your means and living situation.

Food Quality

The quality of the food you eat plays a big role in how well it nourishes and promotes your health. There are many factors to consider concerning the quality of the food you eat:

- Nutrient content
- Cost
- Availability
- Contamination in the form of chemicals, disease causing microbes and heavy metals

When it comes to buying food, better quality food often costs more, but the nutrients obtained per dollar spent also tend to be higher, and the potential for health-damaging contamination tends to be lower.

Food comes from many different sources and there are many variables that can affect its quality:

- Where was it produced?
- Was it factory-farmed or produced on local farms?
- What did it eat before you ate it?
- How long has it been since it was harvested?
- How much has it been processed?

To be in control of your food, you will need to answer these questions and perhaps more. It can take some effort to learn about your food but when it comes to food and health, an ounce of prevention is worth far more than a pound of cure.

Finding Good Food

The best foods are not always available in grocery stores. Therefore you may need to find other sources for your food such as farmer's markets, local farms or even online purchases.

This can be time-consuming, but the gain in food quality and health is worth the effort.

If you eat in a cafeteria, the quality and source of your food will be an unknown.

The best approach in this situation is to make good food choices in the cafeteria and supplement your diet with healthy snacks.

See Getting the Most from Your Cafeteria for more information.

The following terms are commonly used to describe food. They can vary from country to country but here is a layman's summary of information provided by the U.S. Department of Agriculture (www.usda.gov):

Organic

- Products must be grown without the use of synthetic fertilizers, chemicals or sewage sludge and cannot be irradiated or genetically modified.
- Animals can be fed only organic feed (no animal byproducts) and cannot be treated with hormones or antibiotics.
- Animals must have access to the outdoors but do not have to go outdoors to be considered organic.
- There are no organic standards for fish.

Natural or All Natural

- Meat and poultry should not have any added artificial ingredients (such as colors or flavors) or chemical preservatives and should be minimally processed after slaughter.
- Means nothing with regard to how the animal is raised or fed.

GMO

- GMO stands for genetically modified organism, which means that the organism (food) has been genetically altered or gene-spliced to change one or more of its characteristics.
- A food made from a GMO does not have to be labeled as such, which means that consumers can unknowingly buy and consume GMO products. Much of the corn and soy grown in the United States is a GMO.
- Foods that contain no GMO ingredients are sometimes labeled "GMO free" or "Non-GMO".
- GMO foods cannot be labeled as "organic".

No Added Hormones or Hormone Free
- Animals are raised without the use of growth hormones.
- The use of hormones is not permitted in hogs and poultry in the United States.

No Antibiotics or Antibiotic Free
- Animals are raised without the use of antibiotics.

Free Range *(applies only to poultry animals raised for meat)*
- Animals must have some access to the outdoors.
- Animals may spend no time outdoors but as long as there is access to the outdoors, they can be classified as Free Range.
- The access can be as simple as a small door in a warehouse full of thousands of birds that leads to a fenced-in patch of dirt or concrete, or it can be open access to a pasture.

Pasture Raised
- Animals are raised on a pasture rather than in confined facilities or feedlots.

Cage Free
- Animals are not caged, although they may be kept in a confined area such as a large shed or warehouse.

Grass Fed (Grass Finished)
- Animals eat grass from weaning to slaughter
- Does not imply animals are pasture raised, only that their feed is primarily grass.
- Does not mean animals are organic, hormone or antibiotic free.

Grain Fed (Grain Finished)
- Animals are fed a grain product (typically corn and soy, often GMO) to fatten them before slaughter. This technique is common to industrial feedlots and large poultry and hog production facilities.

Below are some general guidelines to help you make more-informed and cost-effective decisions about your food purchases.

ANIMAL AND SEAFOOD PRODUCTS

It is often said that you are what you eat. However, when it comes to cattle, bison, pork, poultry, seafood and eggs, a more appropriate expression is: "You are what you eat, eats."

The reason for this is the nutrient content and the quality of the flesh and fat from animals we consume is highly dependent on what they eat, as well as how the animal is raised and slaughtered.

Ground meat products can be a mix of meat from numerous animals. This mixing can significantly increase the risk of contamination because one sick/contaminated animal can affect many hundreds of pounds of ground meat.

A good practice when buying ground meat is to choose a whole cut and have your butcher trim off the fat and grind it for you.

Cattle, Bison, Sheep
Most red meat available in stores and restaurants comes from animals that have been grass-fed in the early part of their lives and grain-fed in industrial feed lots for the last few months of their lives.

Grain feeding (typically with corn and soy) rapidly fattens the animal in the short period of time just before slaughter.

In addition, growth hormones may be used to boost the weight and muscle mass of the animals. This practice is very common in the

United States and Canada but has been banned by the European Union due to potential human health concerns.

Cattle, bison and sheep are ruminants, meaning they are designed to eat grass. Feeding them grain can significantly alter the nutrient profile of the meat and fat by increasing total saturated fat content and skewing the omega-6 to omega-3 ratio in an unhealthy direction.[1]

Grain feeding can also cause severe digestive problems in ruminants that often require the use of antibiotics to "force" the grain digestive process. This can lead to possible antibiotic contamination of the meat.

Animals that are pasture raised and grass fed throughout their lives (grass-finished) tend to be much healthier, and so is their meat and fat.[2] For example, grass-finished beef:

- Has one-half to one-third the fat of corn-fed beef, and when trimmed can be lower in fat than chicken.
- Has up to 10 times the level of heart-healthy omega-3 fatty acids as corn-fed cattle.
- Has as much as five times the amount of CLA as grain-fed beef. CLA (conjugated linoleic acid) is an omega-3 fatty acid that is thought to reduce the risk of cancer, obesity, diabetes and a number of immune disorders.
- Has up to four times the vitamin E and seven times the beta carotene than grain fed beef (beta carotene is converted by the body into vitamin A).
- Is often raised without the use of antibiotics and hormones.

The bottom line is, just as it is not healthy for cattle, bison and lamb to eat large amounts of grain, it is not very healthy for you to eat grain-fed cattle, bison and lamb.

Unfortunately, pasture raised, grass-finished meat is less available than mass-produced, grain-fed meat and can cost more. However, it does offer significant benefits in terms of health and nutrients per dollar.

An online search for "grass-finished meat" is the best way to find a local supplier. Many will deliver or ship their product frozen. You should sample grass-finished meats before buying a large quantity as the flavor can differ from that of grain-finished meats.

The majority of the beef in the United States comes from grain-finished, feed-lot animals. Unless otherwise labeled, most beef products can contain trace levels of hormones, antibiotics and chemical residues such as pesticides from the feed products.

Bison is now becoming more available in stores. Unless otherwise labeled, it too is grain finished, primarily to change the color of its fat from slightly yellow (when grass finished) to white, which is more what customers expect to see.

Bison meat is naturally leaner and has more protein and iron than a comparable portion of beef. Also, bison are normally raised without the use of hormones and antibiotics. However, similar to beef, the fat from grain-finished bison is less healthy, making grass-finished bison a much healthier choice.

Here are a few things to keep in mind when choosing your beef, bison and lamb meat:

- Organic does not mean grass-finished, only that the meat is free of hormones, antibiotics and chemical residues. Most organic beef, bison and lamb sold in the United States is grain finished.

- Grass-Finished does not mean organic. To carry that designation, the animals must be free of hormones and antibiotics and graze on organic pastures and only be fed organic feed.

- Natural or All Natural means that the meat contains no artificial ingredients and is minimally processed after slaughter. There is no guarantee that a "natural" meat is any healthier for you than one that isn't although from an advertising buzzword perspective, it sure sounds healthier.

BEEF, BISON, AND LAMB QUALITY

Better Quality	Average Quality	Lesser Quality
Organic, pasture raised	All natural	Store brands
Grass finished (local)	Hormone and antibiotic free (typically grain finished so may contain chemical residues from feed)	Pre-frozen patties or cuts
Minimal or no grain feed		Feed-lot, grain finished
Hormone and antibiotic free		May contain hormone, antibiotic and chemical residues
		Canned meat products

Pork

Most modern hog production facilities contain thousands of hogs jammed cheek to jowl in pens that are often so small the animals can't even turn around. They are fed grain-based commercial feed that may or may not contain animal byproducts.

Add to that the antibiotics to treat illness brought on by unsanitary confinement conditions and the lack of anything even resembling the natural environment of a hog, and the pork from these animals can be far from optimum when it comes to promoting health.

Unfortunately, most of the pork products that are readily available in stores, such as bacon, pork chops, ribs, loin-cuts and ham, come from these animals. These pork products may contain antibiotic residues but should be hormone free as the use of growth hormones in hogs is not allowed in the United States

A much healthier meat comes from pastured hogs that forage outdoors and live like a hog should live. These animals eat just about anything they can find such as grass, leaves, grubs, roots, acorns, berries, fruits, eggs, etc. and about anything else they come across in the pastures and woods where they live.

> **Did You Know?**
> - Ham may be fresh, cured,* or cured-and-smoked.
> - Ham is the cured leg of pork.
> - Fresh ham is an uncured leg of pork.
> - Fresh ham will bear the term "fresh" as part of the product name and is an indication that the product is not cured.
> - "Turkey" ham is a ready-to-eat product made from cured thigh meat of turkey.
> - The term "turkey ham" is always followed by the statement "cured turkey thigh meat."
>
> Source: USDA Ham and Food Safety Fact Sheet; April, 2007.
> *Curing is a method of preserving meat, usually with salt, nitrites and/or nitrates.

Just because a hog is pasture raised doesn't mean it is only eating what it finds. Some farmers supplement their hogs' diet with grains, a practice that can alter the quality of the meat and fat, similar to the effects of feeding grain to ruminants.

However, even with moderate grain supplementation, hogs that are pasture raised tend to be much healthier and rarely require the use of antibiotics. Depending on the amount of commercial grain they eat, they are also less likely to be pesticide contaminated.

Many pastured hog producers claim that their hogs are leaner and lower in saturated fat and have higher levels of heart-healthy omega-3, vitamin A and vitamin E than factory-raised hogs. Research to confirm the nutrient content of pastured hog products is still in progress.

Pork Quality

Better Quality	Average Quality	Lesser Quality
Organic, pasture raised	All natural	Store brands
Antibiotic free	Antibiotic free	Pre-frozen ground or cuts
	Usually grain-fed, factory-produced	May contain antibiotic and chemical residues
		Canned meat products

Commercial Packaged Meats

Examples: Bacon, Bologna, Bratwurst, Hams, some Deli Meats, Hot Dogs, Pepperoni, Salami, Sausage, etc.

These highly-processed forms of meat and meat byproducts are inherently unhealthy due to their high fat and sodium content as well as other added chemicals such as preservatives coloring agents and flavor enhancers.

If you choose to eat any of these products, do so rarely and in small quantities.

Chicken and Turkey

Much of the poultry in the United States comes from chickens and turkeys that are raised by the thousands in huge warehouses where:

- The birds live in their own waste and often get sick from breathing the dust and ammonia from their own excrement.
- Bird breeding creates "ready to harvest" birds in as little as 35 days with legs that can barely support their massive body weight.
- Each bird often has less than a half a square foot in which to move and their beaks may be clipped to reduce injuries from fighting in such cramped quarters.
- Antibiotics may be used in the bird's feed to prevent disease from the overcrowded and unhealthy conditions and to spur growth.
- Birds are fed an unnatural diet that may contain poultry and other animal products such as bones, feathers, blood, offal, manure, grease, fishmeal, and diseased animal parts.

Add to that the unsanitary conditions found in many of the huge slaughter houses, and the neatly packaged poultry you buy in your local grocery store has a less-than-healthy shadow upon it.

A healthier choice is meat from chickens and turkeys that are pasture-raised and that eat natural food of insects, worms, grubs and green plants.

As with grass-fed beef, the meat from pasture raised birds tends to be significantly higher in heart-healthy omega-3 fatty acids and lower in overall fat content. Pasture-raised birds tend to be healthier and so is their meat.

Unfortunately, pasture-raised poultry is not commonly available in local stores so you may need to do an online search for a local supplier.

Below are some layman's definitions of terms you will commonly see on packaged poultry products:

- Organic – birds are fed organic food, must have access to the outdoors and are given no antibiotics. Apart from what the birds eat and the limited outdoor access, most are grown and processed in the same way as non-organic birds. The meat from organic birds is not irradiated.

- Natural or All Natural – means the meat is minimally processed after slaughter and is free of artificial ingredients. These birds may have been given antibiotics and may have eaten pesticide contaminated feed.

- Fresh – means the poultry cuts have never been below 26 °F (not frozen hard).

- Free ranging – an ill-defined term that means the birds must have access to the outdoors. Most commonly, the access for thousands of birds is a small door in a warehouse that leads to a little fenced-in patch of dirt or concrete, a reality far from the image created by the term "free-ranging."

- Hormone Free – the U.S. Food and Drug Administration (FDA) does not allow the use of growth hormones in poultry so any label you see advertising hormone-free poultry is simply a ploy to catch the eye of the uninformed consumer.

- Antibiotic Free – means the birds were raised without the use of antibiotics. In recent years some major poultry manufacturers have been limiting the use of antibiotics and are producing antibiotic-free birds.

CHICKEN AND TURKEY QUALITY

Better Quality	Average Quality	Lesser Quality
Organic, pasture-raised	Natural or All Natural	Store brands
Antibiotic free	Antibiotic free	Pre-frozen cuts
Minimal or no grain feed	Typically grain-fed, so meat may contain chemical residues from feed	Warehouse-raised
		May contain antibiotic and chemical residues
		Canned poultry products

Eggs

When chickens are pasture raised and eat their natural food, the eggs they produce are much healthier for you than those from birds that are jammed into cages and fed commercial feed.

One study found that chickens housed indoors and deprived of fresh greens produced eggs that were artificially low in heart-healthy omega-3 fats, and that the eggs from pastured hens can contain 10 times as much omega-3 as indoor birds eating commercial feed.[3]

When the nutrient content of eggs from 14 pastured flocks around the United States was measured and compared to the official U.S.

Department of Agriculture (USDA) nutrient data for commercial eggs, the pastured eggs contained up to:[4]

- 1/3 less cholesterol and 1/4 less saturated fat
- 2/3 more vitamin A and 3 times more vitamin E
- 2 times more omega-3 fatty acids
- 7 times more beta carotene (a vitamin A precursor)

Unless otherwise labeled, most of the eggs available in stores are from caged birds that are fed commercial feed. Many stores now offer more costly specialty eggs but the labels on those products can be confusing and sometimes deceptive:

- Cage-Free – means that unlike caged birds, the birds can move around and lay eggs in nests. It does not mean the birds go outdoors or are pasture fed. Cage-free birds are often kept in huge warehouses crammed full of thousands of birds.
- Free Range – there is no regulation concerning what this means for egg producing birds.
- Grain Fed – is used on egg packaging to entice consumers who do not know the natural diet of chickens. The advantage of grain-fed birds can be that these birds are not fed any animal, fish or shellfish byproducts. The disadvantage is the birds are not eating their natural food.
- Organic – means the birds are fed with organic feed (no additive, animal by-products or GMO). The hens must also live cage free, have access to the outdoors and be treated with high animal-welfare standards. The advantage of organic eggs is they are mostly free of contaminants.

The first three descriptors are encompassed in the "organic" designation, so you might as well buy organic if you are going to buy specialty eggs. Organic eggs cost more than cheap, store-brand eggs, but in terms of potential health benefits, they are worth it.

Clearly, the best eggs are those from a local farm that pastures its birds and allows them to forage and eat their natural food. However, availability of these eggs is often limited.

Farmers markets can be a source of pastured eggs or an online search can often reveal a local supplier. Eggs are such a health-building food that a little effort put into obtaining top quality eggs is easily justified.

Cafeteria eggs are often pre-blended with a preservative and delivered in a 5-gallon dispenser box. The quality of these egg products is typically very low.

EGG QUALITY

Better Quality	Average Quality	Lesser Quality
Eggs from pastured birds eating mostly foraged food Organic (farm or store purchased)	Cage free Grain fed	Inexpensive store brands Liquid form of eggs or egg whites in a carton

Fish and Seafood

Fish and shellfish from ocean and freshwater sources are very often contaminated at some level with heavy metals, such as mercury. Chemicals such as polychlorinated biphenyls (PCBs), chlordane, dioxins and DDT are other possible contaminants.

A 2009 U.S. Environmental Protection Agency study revealed that all of the fish taken from the 500 lakes and reservoirs across the United States had mercury and PCB contamination. Other contaminants, such as dioxins, were also frequently found.[5]

The more polluted the water, the more polluted the fish or shellfish that lives in it. Therefore, it is advised that you ask those handling the fish where it comes from so you can make a more informed decision.

Smaller fish, such as anchovies, mackerel and sardines, are lower on the food chain and tend to be the least contaminated. These fish grow quickly and don't accumulate toxins as much as bigger fish, such as shark, swordfish, king mackerel and tilefish.

There is a great deal of controversy about how much and what type of fish and shellfish is safe to eat. Here is a shortened version of the guidelines from the U.S. Environmental Protection Agency (www.epa.gob/fishadvisories/advice/).

For children and pregnant women:

- Avoid eating shark, swordfish, king mackerel, or tilefish – due to high levels of mercury.
- Consume up to 12 ounces per week of fish and shellfish that are lower in mercury such as:
    o Shrimp, canned light tuna, salmon, pollock, and catfish.
    o Consumption of albacore tuna should be limited to six ounces per week due to higher levels of mercury than canned light tuna.
- If the source of locally caught fish is unknown, limit consumption to six ounces per week and don't consume any other fish during that week.

It is beyond the scope of this book to address all of the benefits and health issues associated with fish and shellfish consumption. At Nutrition Coaches, LLC we recommend that you:

- Stay well within the above EPA guidelines when consuming fish and shellfish.

- Be very cautious of mercury contamination from fish and shellfish consumption whether you are young, pregnant or not.

- Choose wild-caught over farmed salmon. Virtually all Atlantic salmon is now farmed. Farmed salmon is often labeled "color-added."

- Choose small fish over large fish (for example, choose sardines over tuna and chunk light tuna over albacore tuna).

- Avoid fresh water fish from unknown waters.

- Be wary of any fish or seafood product that is labeled as "organic." The USDA currently has no organic standards for seafood.

- If pregnant or breast feeding, be extra cautious about your fish and seafood consumption due to mercury contamination and its effects on fetal development.

MERCURY LEVELS IN COMMON FISH AND SHELLFISH*

Low	Moderate	High
Catfish	Bass	Bluefish
Salmon	Cod	Grouper
Sardine	Halibut	Shark
Scallops	Mahi Mahi	Swordfish
Shrimp	Snapper	Tilefish
Trout	Tuna, chunk light	Tuna, albacore

*Data from US Food and Drug Administration and from Environmental Working Group (www.EWG.org)

The Environmental Working Group (www.ewg.org) is an excellent resource to learn more about fish and shellfish contamination and consumption guidelines. This is one area where it is well worth your time to investigate the benefits and dangers associated with seafood products.

Produce

Evidence is beginning to emerge that organic produce has higher nutrient content than conventionally grown produce.[6] Many people also report that organic fruits and vegetables taste better, although this may be a consequence of freshness as organic produce is usually locally produced and spends less time in transit than commercial produce.

Another benefit of organic produce is that it contains far lower levels of contaminants, such as pesticides, which may cause lasting damage to human health, particularly during fetal development and early childhood.[7]

The downside is that buying organic produce can be expensive and may not always be available in your local supermarket.

Fortunately, some produce can be purchased in non-organic form as it is not as heavily pesticide contaminated.

The Environmental Working Group (www.ewg.org) has published a guide that identifies the 12 most contaminated produce items (Dirty Dozen) that should be bought organic and 15 items that have minimal pesticide contamination (Clean 15).

They are:

Dirty Dozen (buy these organic)

1. Celery
2. Peaches
3. Strawberries
4. Apples
5. Blueberries
6. Nectarines
7. Bell Peppers
8. Spinach
9. Kale
10. Cherries
11. Potatoes
12. Grapes (imported)

Clean 15

1. Onions
2. Avocado
3. Sweet Corn
4. Pineapple
5. Mangos
6. Sweet Peas
7. Asparagus
8. Kiwi
9. Cabbage
10. Eggplant
11. Cantaloupe
12. Watermelon
13. Grapefruit
14. Sweet Potato
15. Honeydew Melon

A handy, printable pocket guide that contains this information can easily be downloaded at: www.foodnews.org.

In general, you are better off purchasing produce grown locally rather than that grown in places where pesticide and fertilizer may be unregulated. In addition, the longer produce is off the plant, the more the nutrient value is diminished.

Choose local sources such as farmers markets for fresher, more nutritious produce.

What is a PLU?

Produce in grocery stores is often labeled with a four or five digit PLU code (price look-up code) that is used by the cashier to identify the food and speed-up the checkout process.

Conventionally raised produce has a 4-digit PLU code.

Organic produce has a 5-digit PLU code that begins with the number 9.

Genetically modified (GMO) produce has a 5-digit PLU code that begins with the number 8.

Examples:
- 4011 = conventional banana
- 94011 = organic banana
- 84011 = genetically modified banana

High quality frozen produce can also be an okay choice as the blanching process just prior to freezing can lock in many nutrients. Consumption of canned fruits and vegetables should be minimized because of potential leaching of BPA from the lining of the can.[8]

Organic or not, all produce should be thoroughly washed before eating. The use of a commercial vegetable/fruit wash is recommended. You can also make your own wash by adding two tablespoons of distilled white vinegar to a pint of water.

Dairy

Dairy products are a major part of the modern diet, with people consuming milk, cheese, yoghurt and ice cream several times per day. Dairy products can also be found in baked goods, chocolate, processed deli meats, cereals, protein powders and energy bars.

Government agencies and dairy producers spend immense amounts of money promoting the consumption of milk and milk products – the government for claims of health – the dairy industry for profit.

This dairy advertising campaign has been so effective that many people now believe that drinking milk is indispensable for the growth of strong bones and health.

That is wrong.

Cow's milk is a food that is naturally designed to support the health and growth of baby cows. In some parts of the world, it has been used as human food for many centuries. In other places, dairy was never a part of the local diet.

> **It is hard to imagine that humans can only be healthy if they drink the milk of another species. If consuming dairy was essential to forming strong bones and maintaining health, those who lived in areas where dairy was not available would not have survived.**

Therefore, it is reasonable to conclude that if dairy "works" for you (see Food Sensitivity in Section IV) you can eat it in moderation and be healthy. If dairy does not "work" for you, you can eat a balanced dairy-free diet and still be healthy.

If you do consume dairy products, quality is very important. For example, the use of hormones to stimulate milk production in cows is a common practice in the United States Traces of these hormones can be passed on to those who drink the milk or eat concentrated milk products such as cheese.

The health effects of these hormones, even in trace amounts, are still being studied. Some experts believe these hormones play a role in promoting the development of breast and colon cancer, premature growth stimulation in infants, and development of abnormally large mammary glands in young children.[9,10]

The evidence of possible health effects from a hormone commonly used in the United States, called Bovine Growth Hormone (BGH), was sufficient for Canada and the European Union to ban its use. The hormone is still approved for use in the United States

To limit your exposure to hormones, antibiotics and other chemicals, choose organic dairy products over less expensive non-organic milk products. Another option is to buy from a local source that supplies hormone-free milk.

It is unlikely that you will have organic dairy products available to you in a cafeteria so apply moderation when consuming dairy products in that setting.

Organic dairy products will cost more than non-organic, but this is one area where a dollar saved is not worth the risk.

SEEDS AND TREE NUTS

Seeds and tree nuts, such as almonds, pecans and walnuts, are a very healthy food when eaten in moderation. They make a convenient and satisfying snack because of their rich flavor and relatively high protein and fat content.

However, the more seeds and tree nuts are processed, such as by roasting at high temperatures, the less healthy they become due to the damaging effects of heat on the natural oils in the nut or seed. Therefore, it is best to consume nuts and seeds in raw form or in the least processed form possible.

Pesticide contamination of nuts and seeds can also be a problem. According to the Pesticide Action Network Database (www.pesticideinfo.org), more than 19 million pounds of chemicals and pesticides were used on the 2008 California almond crop alone.

For health reasons, you should choose organic sources for nuts and seeds whenever possible.

Store all nuts, seeds and their butters in the refrigerator even if "no refrigeration required" appears on the label.

Peanuts

Peanuts are actually not a nut but a bean that grows in the ground. Like tree nuts, they are subject to contamination and when possible you should choose organic.

Peanuts are susceptible to growing mold, particularly if they are improperly stored. A mold common to peanuts can produce a toxin called "aflatoxin." This toxin can also be found on corn and other grains.

According to research available at the U.S. National Institute of Health, acute and chronic exposure to aflatoxin has been associated with liver cancer.[11] The good news is that raw peanuts are lot-tested in the United States to ensure aflatoxin levels stay within safe limits.

Most commercial peanut butter available in grocery stores is made from non-organic peanuts and contains large amounts of sugar and hydrogenated or partially-hydrogenated oils.

For this reason, you should choose a peanut butter that has only the following ingredients:

- Peanuts (preferably organic)
- Peanut oil
- Salt or sea salt

If you do not have organic peanut products available in your local store, they can be purchased online and delivered at a very reasonable cost.

Mold growth is less likely at cold temperatures so you should store all peanuts and peanut butter in the refrigerator, even if "refrigeration not needed" appears on the label.

Some stores offer grind-your-own peanut butter. However, without knowing the freshness of the peanuts or how long they have been sitting in the storage bin, you are better off choosing a sealed, prepackaged product.

GRAINS AND BREADS

According to the U.S. Food and Drug Administration, "whole grains" consist of the intact, ground, cracked or flaked fruit of the grains whose principal components – the starchy endosperm, germ and bran – are present in the same relative proportions as they exist in the intact grain.

Examples of whole grains are:

- Barley
- Buckwheat
- Corn
- Oats
- Quinoa
- Rice
- Rye
- Wheat
- Wild and brown rice

In contrast, products made from refined grains, such as white flour, are missing the two most nutritious and fiber-rich parts of the grain seed: the outside bran layer and the germ.

White flour has a longer shelf life and makes fluffier breads and pastries but is virtually devoid of natural nutrients. That is why white flour is often "enriched" by adding in minimal amounts of B vitamins and iron to make up for the natural nutrients destroyed by processing.

When you eat "white" products, such as white bread, they are rapidly turned into sugar and cause blood sugar imbalances that can trigger energy crashes and body fat storage. White rice will have a similar effect as will many breakfast cereals, crackers and baked goods.

Quinoa

Quinoa (pronounced keen-wah) is a nutritious grain that is high in protein and fiber. It is gluten-free, easily digested and can be used in place of rice or pasta.

To cook quinoa, add one part quinoa to two parts water, stir, cover and cook until all the water is absorbed (10 to 15 minutes). It has a slight nut-like flavor and can be served as a side dish, in soups or salads, as a pilaf, in a stir fry or even as a breakfast cereal.

For additional flavor, broth or vegetable stock can be used in place of the water during cooking. In the United States, quinoa can be found in most natural food stores and in the natural food section of some grocery stores. It can also be purchased online.

It is best to avoid eating non whole-grain products. If you do, keep the quantity small and compliment with nutritious whole foods.

When shopping, be wary of deceptive labeling. A label that reads "made with whole grain" just means that some whole grains exist in the product. How much is not clear.

A "multi-grain" label means that the product was made from several different grains. It may or may not contain any "whole" grain.

When buying bread, look for "100% Whole Grain" on the label. The bread will tend to be less rubbery and heavier than that made from white flour. The same approach applies to buying cereal.

When buying rice, choose brown or wild rice over white.

Food Preparation, Handling and Storage

Once you get your food home, how you handle, store and prepare it is important from both a food safety and nutrient benefit perspective. Some basic concepts are provided in the following Web site maintained by the U.S. Department of Health and Human Services: www.foodsafety.gov. The site is easy to use, informative and well worth a visit.

Below are some additional tips and ideas to help keep your food safe and minimize nutrient loss:

- Save time by preparing raw and fast-cooking foods while slower foods cook.

- If meat/poultry/fish and vegetables and fruits will be cut on the same cutting board, cut the fruits and vegetables first to prevent contamination from the raw animal products.

- Do not allow utensils, containers, wrappings or plates that have been in contact with raw flesh products to contact the finished cooked product.

Meats, Poultry, Fish

- Refrigerate all meats and fish.

- Whole cuts of meat should be broiled, grilled, roasted or baked. Frying is a less healthy way to cook meat.

- If you fry meat, such as a ground meat patty, cook it at a low temperature and flip it often to minimize charring or burning, which can create carcinogenic (cancer causing) substances.[12]

> **Cooking for Yourself**
>
> Try stir frying. It is a fast, easy way to cook a variety of tasty foods. And the best part, there is only one pan to clean.
>
> Is making a salad for one a hassle? Try making three nights worth of salad and store it in the refrigerator. Then, tired or not, you will have a ready-to-eat salad waiting for you each night.

Fruits and Vegetables

- Keep fruits and vegetables separate as some fruits emit a gas that can speed up the ripening of nearby produce. To speed up ripening, put a banana or apple in a closed paper bag with the fruit or produce you want to ripen.

- Store in the refrigerator:

    o Apples and ripe avocados can be stored unwrapped.

    o Berries, grapes, peaches and nectarines should be stored in a perforated bag.

    o Artichokes, asparagus, bell peppers, carrots, cherries, broccoli, Brussels sprouts cauliflower, cabbage, celery, cucumbers, peas, summer squash, etc. can be stored in a plastic bag.

    o Washed green beans, lettuce and leafy greens should be shaken or spun dry and stored in a plastic bag with a paper towel to absorb excess moisture.

- Store potatoes, onions and garlic bulbs unwrapped in a cool, dry, dark place.

- Store apricots, bananas, citrus, kiwis, melons, papayas, peaches, pears, pineapple, plums and tomatoes at room temperature in a bowl and out of direct sunlight. Keep bananas away from ripe fruit.

- Avoid soaking vegetables for more than a few minutes as nutrients can leach out of them.

- Avoid overcooking vegetables as that can reduce their nutrient content. Vegetables, such as broccoli, should have a slight crunch after cooking.

- Steaming or stir-frying vegetables is preferred to boiling for preserving nutrient content.

- If you boil vegetables, add them to the pot after the water has come to a boil and use the left-over water to cook rice or in a soup, sauce or stew.

- When stir frying, use minimum cooking oil. A small amount of water added to a covered, hot pan will flash into steam and speed the cooking. If more oil is desired for flavor or texture, add it just before you are done cooking the vegetables to minimize overheating it.

- Keep skins on for cooking and if desired, remove them afterwards.

> **Preserving Nutrients**
>
> A clever way to retain vegetable nutrients is to use the steam from cooking rice to steam your vegetables.
>
> To do this, put your vegetables in a pot-top steamer on top of the rice pot. Then, any minerals that leach out of the vegetables during steaming will be absorbed by the rice below.
>
> You will also save energy by using only one stove burner to cook two items.

Cookware

Many pots, pans, utensils and bakeware are now made with non-stick coatings. The cooking and clean-up benefits of non-stick cookware are terrific but there is some question about the safety of these coatings, especially when heated to high temperatures.

One concern is the release of PFC's (polyfluoroalkyl chemicals) from non-stick coatings into the food or air. It has been known for decades that fumes released from overheating certain types of non-stick pans can be fatal to pet birds, and can cause flu-like symptoms in humans.[13]

There is ongoing debate concerning the possible human health effects of PFCs but the growing body of evidence linking PFC exposure to health issues such as cancers, hypothyroidism, immune system problems, reproductive abnormalities and birth defects is enough to suggest that minimizing exposure to these chemicals is prudent.[14]

PFC's are used in many household products, and whether or not non-stick cookware is a primary path of PFC contamination remains unclear. However, contamination is an issue as 95 percent of Americans now have measureable levels of PFC in their blood.[15]

If you use non-stick coated cookware, cook at low temperatures and avoid overheating it. Start your cooking process on low heat settings as it only takes a minute or two for a pan to reach "toxic" temperatures when preheated on a hot burner.

The use of more traditional cookware, such as cast iron, stainless steel, glass or enamel cookware is a safer, PFC-free option.

Microwave Cooking

The speed at which microwave ovens heat food makes them very convenient. This rapid heating is accomplished by focusing a large amount of microwave energy directly into the food.

Whether or not microwave energy is a safe and healthy way to cook remains a subject of debate. Some say it alters the food molecules into an unhealthy, cancer-causing state and destroys the nutrient content of food. Others argue that it does nothing more to food than traditional cooking and can actually preserve the nutrient content of food.

Unfortunately, there is little scientific evidence available from which to draw a firm conclusion. A reasonable approach is to err on the side of caution and stick with time-proven conventional cooking techniques until the issue is resolved by further research.

If you do microwave your food, be aware that chemicals can leach from plastic containers, lids and wraps commonly used in microwave cooking. Containers labeled "microwave-safe" are not necessarily chemical-free.

> **Microwave Popcorn**
>
> Popcorn is a popular snack, particularly in college dormitories. Unfortunately, the packaging used in some commercial microwavable brands can leach chemicals into the popcorn and may also release fumes that are known to cause respiratory health issues.[16]
>
> With that in mind, here is a simple and inexpensive way to microwave popcorn with little risk of chemical contamination:
>
> - Mix ¼ cup of popcorn kernels (about a handful) with a teaspoon virgin olive oil (optional) and 1 teaspoon of salt (or salt to taste later).
> - Place the kernel mixture in the bottom of a brown paper lunch bag. (A large glass bowl covered with a plate can also work)
> - Fold and seal the top of the bag with a single staple and microwave on High for 2 to 3 minutes.
> - Add seasoning as desired.

One chemical of note is BPA (Bisphenol-A), and in particular, the effect of BPA on babies fed with plastic or plastic-lined baby bottles and on children.

According to the FDA:

> **"Recent studies provide reason for some concern about the potential effects of BPA on the brain, behavior, and prostate gland of fetuses, infants and children."[17]**

And while the FDA supports steps to reduce human exposure to BPA and is pursuing additional studies on the safety of BPA, several countries and a handful of states have already banned the sale of baby bottles that contain BPA.

It is probably only a matter of time before all plastic food and drink containers will be required to be BPA free, but until then, be smart and steer clear of BPA contamination by using microwave-safe glass or ceramic containers instead of plastic when microwaving your food.

SECTION VII

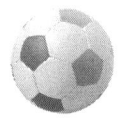

FEED THE CHAMPION IN YOU

There is a champion in everyone. Sometimes it is the least expected player who scores a great goal at a crucial time or makes an incredible goal-line stand or rises to lead when all others fail. A champion can appear at any time in any endeavor, not just soccer or sport.

But the opportunity to be champion won't wait for you to get ready. You have to be ready when it arrives. For as quickly as opportunity appears, it can depart just as fast.

Being ready for every opportunity life throws your way is what eating well is all about. Your *Soccer Nutrition Handbook* has provided you with the tools needed to eat well. All you have to do is patiently incorporate that information into your everyday life.

You know that regularly eating nutritious food is essential to maintaining health. You also know that your soccer performance is powered by everything you eat and drink, and that properly fueling your body on a daily basis is the best way to ensure you are ready to play one of the world's most demanding games.

You also now know that nutrition is not an event or a one-day activity. Nutrition is a path, a path of learning that you move along each day of your life. How you walk that path is completely up to you. It is your body, it is your life and it is your soccer performance.

Skill training can make you clever on the field.

Tactical training can make you smarter on the field.

Fitness training can make you stronger on the field.

But if you come up short in the nutrition department, you can train and train and train and still end up far below where your hard work should have taken you.

Here are the some of the key elements that you have learned:

- One size does not fit all when it comes to nutrition.
- Take control of your food.
- Minimize consumption of sweets.
- Eat more real food and less industrial food.
- Learn which foods work best for your individual genetic makeup.
- Listen to what your body tells you about your food.
- Balance portions of your ideal foods for optimum daily energy.
- Hydrate properly throughout your soccer season.
- Use appropriate supplements only as needed and always honor the purity of sport.
- Maintain safe and healthy levels of body fat.
- Address health and digestive issues that can affect performance.
- Make smart food choices to limit unhealthy fats and food contaminants.

Follow these fundamental concepts and you will be your own nutrition expert. Others will try to tell you what is best for you. Hear what they say but always listen to your own body first when it comes to nutrition. You know better than anyone else what works for you.

As you age and change, your nutritional needs can also change. Go with the flow and adjust what you eat accordingly.

Food wisdom has always been the key to survival. It is only in recent history that food has been taken for granted, and food wisdom has become mired in ignorance.

Become food wise among those who are not and you will rise above your competition. Food is one of life's wonders. Understand food and never take it for granted for it truly forms the rungs of every ladder you will climb to success.

**If you properly feed the champion in you,
you will be a champion!**

REFERENCES

SECTION I

1. Appleton, N. *Lick the Sugar Habit.* New York: Avery/Penguin Group, Inc., 1996.

2. Johnson, R.K., Appel, L.J., Brands, M., Howard, B.V., Lefevre, M., Lustig, R.H., Sacks, F., Steffen, L.M., and Wylie-Rosett, J. Dietary sugars intake and cardiovascular health: a scientific statement from the American Heart Association. *Journal of the American Heart Association Circulation,* 2009; 120:1011-1020.

3. Blaylock, R.L. *Excitotoxins: The Taste That Kills.* New Mexico: Health Press, 1997.

4. Swithers, S.E., and Davidson, T.L. A role for sweet taste: calorie predictive relations in energy regulation by rats. *Behavioral Neuroscience,* 2008; 122:161-173.

5. Avena, N.M., Rada, P., and Hoebel, B.G. Evidence for sugar addiction: behavioral and neurochemical effects of intermittent, excessive sugar intake. *Neuroscience and Biobehavioral Reviews,* 2008; 32.1:20-39.

6. Price, W.A. *Nutrition and Physical Degeneration.* California: The Price-Pottenger Nutrition Foundation, Inc., 2000.

7. Kris-Etherton, P.M., Hecker, K.D., Bonanome, A., Coval, S.M., Binkoski, A.E., Hilpert, K.F., Griel, A.E., and Etherton, T.D. Bioactive compounds in foods: their role in the prevention of cardiovascular disease and cancer. *American Journal of Medicine,* 2002; 113:71S-88S.

8. Potter, J. D., Steinmetz, K. Vegetables, fruit and phytoestrogens as preventive agents. *International Agency for Research on Cancer Scientific Publications,* 1996; 139:61-90.

9. Steinmetz, K., Potter, J. D. Vegetables, fruit, and cancer. II. Mechanisms. *Cancer Causes Control.* 1991; Nov. 2.6:427-442.

10. Watson, George. *Nutrition and Your Mind.* New York: Bantam Books, 1974.

11. Wiley, R.A. BioBalance: *The Acid/Alkaline Solution to the Food-Mood-Health Puzzle.* Utah: Essential Science Publishing, 2002.

12. Wiley, R.A. BioBalance2: *Achieving Optimum Health Through Acid/Alkaline Nutrition.* Utah: Essential Science Publishing, 2002.

13. Wolcott, William and Fahey, T. *The Metabolic Typing Diet.* New York: Broadway Books, 2002.

Section II

1. Pichan, G., Gauttam, R.K., Tomar, O.S., and A.C. Bajaj. Effects of primary hypohydration on physical work capacity. *International Journal of Biometeorology,* 1988; 32.1:176-180.

2. Walsh, R.M., Noakes, T.D., Hawley, J.A., and Dennis, S.C. Impaired high-intensity cycling performance time at low levels of dehydration. *International Journal of Sports Medicine,* 1994; 15:392-398.

3. Kenney, L.W. Dietary water and sodium requirements for active adults. *Sports Science Exchange 92,* 2004; 17.1.

4. American College of Sports Medicine. *American College of Sports Medicine Clarifies Indicators for Fluid Replacement.* ACSM News Releases, February 2004, available at: http://www.acsm.org. Accessed August 4, 2010.

5. MayoClinic. *Water: How Much Should You Drink Every Day?* Available at: http://www.mayoclinic.com/health/water/NU00283. Accessed November 3, 2009.

6. Casa, D.J., Armstrong, L.E., Hillman, S.K., Montain, S.J., Reiff, R.V., Rich, B.S.E., Roberts, W.O., and Stone, J.A. National Athletic Trainers' Association position statement: fluid replacement for athletes. *Journal of Athletic Training,* 2000; 35.2:212-224.

7. Williams, Clyde and Nicholas, C.W. Nutrition needs for team sport. *Sports Science Exchange 70,* 1998; 11.3.

8. McGovern, V., Polycarbonate plastics and human BPA exposure: urinary levels rise with use of drinking bottles. *Environmental Health Perspectives,* 2009, 117.9: doi:10.1289/ehp.117-a406b.

9. Keri, R.A., Ho, S-M, Hunt, P.A., Knudsen, K./E., Soto, A.M., Prins, G.S., An evaluation of evidence for the carcinogenic activity of bisphenol A. *Reproductive Toxicology,* 2007; 24.2:240-252.

10. Lang, I.A., Galloway, T.S., Scarlett, A., Henley, W.E., Depledge, M, Wallace, R. B., Melzer, D., Association of urinary bisphenol A concentration with medical disorders and laboratory abnormalities in adults. *Journal of the American Medical Association*, 2008; 300.11:1303-1310.

11. Vom Saal, F.S., Myers, J.P. Bisphenol A and risk of metabolic disorders. *Journal of the American Medical Association*, 2008; 300.11:1353-1355.

12. VanDenBergh, A.J., Houtman, S., Arend, H., Rehrer, N.J., VanDenBoogert, H.J., Oeseburg, B., and Hopman, M.T.E. Muscle glycogen recovery after exercise during glucose and fructose intake monitored by 13C-NMR. *Journal of Applied Physiology*, 1996; 81.4:1495-1500.

13. Jeukendrup, A. Carbohydrate supplementation during exercise: does it help? How much is too much? *Sports Science Exchange 106*, 2007; 20.3.

SECTION III

1. Williams, M.H. Dietary supplements and sports performance: introduction and vitamins. *Journal of the International Society of Sports Nutrition*, 2004; 1.2:1-6

2. Benardot D, et al.: Can vitamin supplements improve sport performance? *Sports Science Exchange Roundtable 2001*; 12.3:1-4.

3. Pauling, Linus, and Cameron, E. *Cancer and Vitamin C*. Philadelphia: Amino Books, Inc., 1979.

4. Hathcock, J.N., Azzi, A., Blumberg, J., Bray, T., Dickinson, A., Frei, B., Jialal, I., Johnston, C.S., Kelly, F.J., Kraemer, K., Packer, L., Parthasarathy, S., Sies, H., and Traber, M.G. Vitamins E and C are safe across a broad range of intakes. *American Journal of Clinical Nutrition*, 2005; 81.4:736-745.

5. Klenner, F.R. Observations on the dose and administration of ascorbic acid when employed beyond the range of a vitamin in human pathology. *Journal of Applied Nutrition*, 1971; 23.3 & 23.4.

6. Holick, M.F. Vitamin D deficiency, medical progress. *The New England Journal of Medicine*, 2007; 357:266-281.

Section IV

1. Tanaka, H., Monahan, K.D., and Seals, D.R. Age-predicted maximal heart rate revisited. *Journal of the American College of Cardiology*, 2001; 37.1:153-156.

2. Andre, F., Andre, C., Colin, L., Cacaraci, F., and Cavagna, S. Role of new allergens and of allergens consumption in the increased incidence of food sensitizations in France. *Toxicology*, 1994; 93:77-83.

3. Branum, A. M., and Lukacs, S.L. Food allergy among U.S. children: trends in prevalence and hospitalizations. *U.S. Dept. of Health and Human Services: National Center for Health Statistics Data Brief*, 2008; 10.10:1-7.

4. Plummer, N. The unseen epidemic: the linked syndromes of achlorhydria and atrophic gastritis. *Townsend Letter for Doctors and Patients*. July, 2004.

5. Bray, G.W. The hypochlorhydria of asthma in childhood. *Quarterly Journal of Medicine*, 1931; 24:181-97.

Section V

1. Clifton, P.M., Keogh, J.B., and Noakes, M., Trans fatty acids in adipose tissue and the food supply are associated with myocardial infarction. *Journal of Nutrition*, 2004; 134.4:874-879.

2. Naruszewicz, M., Daniewski, M., Nowicka, G., Kozlowska-Wojciechowska, M., Trans-unsaturated fatty acids and acrylamide in food as potential atherosclerosis progression factors: based on own studies. *Acta Microbiologica Polonica*, 2003; 52 Suppl:75-81.

3. Mozaffarian, D., Pischon, T., Hankinson, S.E., Rifai, N., Joshipura, K., Willett, W.C., and Rimm, E.B. Dietary intake of trans fatty acids and systemic inflammation in women. *American Journal of Clinical Nutrition*, 2004; 79.4:606-612.

4. Sundram, K., Ismail, A., Hayes, K.C., Jeyamalar, R., and Pathmanathan, R. Trans (elaidic) fatty acids adversely affect the lipoprotein profile relative to specific saturated fatty acids in humans. *Journal of Nutrition*, 1997; 127.3:514S-520S.

5. Pietinen, P., Ascherio, A., Korhonen, P., Harman, A.M., Willett, W.C., Albanes, D., and Virtamo, J. Intake of fatty acids and risk of coronary heart disease in a cohort of Finnish men: the alpha-tocopherol, beta-carotene cancer prevention study. *American Journal of Epidemiology*, 1997; 145.10:876-887.

6. Cancer Research Foundation of America. *Trans Fatty Acids Linked to Breast Cancer Risk*. Available at: http://www.dldewey.com/columns/breast2.htm. Accessed June 28, 2010.

7. Taubes, G., *Good Calories, Bad Calories*. New York: Anchor Books, 2008.

8. Erasmus, U., *Fats that Heal Fats that Kill*. Summertown, TN: Alive Books 1993.

9. Simopoulos, A.P. Evolutionary aspects of omega-3 fatty acids in the food supply. *Prostaglandins, Leukotrienes and Essential Fatty Acids*, 1999; 60: 421-429.

10. Bland, J.S., Costarella, L., Levin, B., et al. Clinical Nutrition – A Functional Approach. Washington: *The Institute for Functional Medicine*, 2004.

11. Daley, C.A., Abbott, A., Doyle, P.S., Nader, G.A., and Larson, S. A review of fatty acid profiles and antioxidant content in grass-fed and grain-fed beef. Nutrition Journal, 2010; 9.10:1-12.

12. Long, Cheryl, and Alterman, T. Meet real free-range eggs. Mother Earth News, 2007; 10/11:1-5.

13. Simopoulos, Artemis P., and Salem, Norman, Jr. Egg yolk as a source of long-chain polyunsaturated fatty acids in infant feeding. American Journal of Clinical Nutrition,1992; 55:411-4.

Section VI

1. Cordain, L., Watkins, B.A., Florant, G.L., Kelher, M., Rogers, L., and Y Li. Fatty acid analysis of wild ruminant tissues: evolutionary implications for reducing diet-related chronic disease. European Journal of Clinical Nutrition, 2002; 56:181-191.

2. Daley, C.A., Abbott, A., Doyle, P.S., Nader, G.A., and Larson, S. A review of fatty acid profiles and antioxidant content in grass-fed and grain-fed beef. *Nutrition Journal*, 2010; 9.10:1-12.

3. Lopez-Bote, C. H., Arias, R.S., Rey, A.I., Castano, A., Isabel, B., Thos, J. Effect of free range feeding on omega 3 fatty acids and alpha tocopherol content and oxidative stability of eggs. *Animal Feed Science and Technology*, 1998; 72:33-40.

4. Long, Cheryl, and Alterman, T. Meet real free-range eggs. *Mother Earth News*, 2007; 10/11:1-5.

5. Environmental Protection Agency. *National Lake Fish Tissue Study*. Available at www.epa.gov/waterscience/fishstudy/. Published September 2009; accessed August 1, 2010.

6. Worthington, V. Nutritional quality of organic versus conventional fruits, vegetables and grains. *The Journal of Alternative and Complementary Medicine*, 2001; 7:161-73.

7. Curl, C., Fenske, R., and Elgethun, K. Organophosphorus pesticide exposure of urban and suburban preschool children with organic and conventional diets. *Environmental Health Perspectives*, 2003; 111.3:377-382.

8. Environmental Working Group. *Canned food test results*. Available at: http://www.ewg.org. Published May 23, 2007; accessed July 30, 2010.

9. Cancer Prevention Coalition. New Study Warns of Breast and Colon Cancer Risks from rBGH Milk. Press Release, Press Conference, National Press Club Washington D.C., January 23, 1996. Available at: http://www.preventcancer.com/press/conference/jan23_96.htm. Accessed May 28, 2010.

10. Epstein, S.S. Potential public health hazards of biosynthetic milk hormones. *International Journal of Health Services,* 1990; 20.1:73-84.

11. National Institute of Environmental Health Sciences. *Aflatoxin and Liver Cancer.* November 2007. Available at: http://www.niehs.nih.gov/health/impacts/aflatoxin.cfm. Accessed July 21, 2010.

12. Anderson, K.E., Sinha, R., Kulldorff, M., Gross, M., Lang, N.P., Barber, C., Harnack, L., DeMagno, E., Bliss, R., Kadlubar, F.F. Meat intake and cooking techniques: associations with pancreatic cancer. *Mutation Research/Fundamental and Molecular Mechanisms of Mutagenesis,* 2002; 506/507:225-231.

13. Environmental Working Group. *Canaries in the kitchen: a Teflon toxicosis.* Available at http://www.ewg.org. Published May 14, 2003; accessed August 13, 2010.

14. Environmental Working Group. *PFC health concerns.* Available at http://www.ewg.org. Published April 3, 2003; accessed August 16, 2010.

15. Environmental Working Group. *PFOA is a pervasive pollutant in human blood, as are other PFC's.* Available at http://www.ewg.org. Published April 3, 2003; accessed August 16, 2010.

16. Rosati, J.A., Krebs, K.A., and Liu, X. Emissions from cooking microwave popcorn. *Critical Reviews in Food Science and Nutrition,* 2007; 47.8:701-709

17. U.S. Food and Drug Administration. *Update on Bisphenol A for use in food contact applications.* Available at http://www.fda.gov. Published January, 2010; accessed August 9, 2010.

APPENDIX

Contents

Diet Plan 1 – Daily Foods
Diet Plan 2 – Daily Foods
Meal Evaluation Form

Additional copies of the Meal Evaluation Form and Diet Plans can be downloaded for free at:

www.NutritionCoaches.com

DIET PLAN 1 – DAILY FOODS

Meat / Fish	Vegetables	Fruits
Light and white meats: Chicken breast Cornish hen Pork, lean Chops and ham Turkey breast Light and white fish: Bass Cod Flounder Halibut Mahi-mahi Sole Snapper` Tuna (light)	Beet Broccoli Brussels sprouts Cabbage Cucumber Pepper (bell, all colors) Radish Potato/yam Sprouts Squash All leafy greens	Apple Apricot Banana Berries Cherries Grapefruit Grapes Kiwi Mango Melon Nectarine Orange Papaya Peach Pear Pineapple Plum Pomegranate Tangerine

	Beans*	
	Garbanzo Navy Pinto White *avoid eating beans with meat	

Grains	Nuts / Seeds*	Fats / Oils*
Whole grain breads Whole grain cereals Barley Buckwheat Cornmeal Oat/Oatmeal Quinoa Rice: Basmati, Brown, Wild Rye Wheat	All *best if consumed in smaller quantities	Butter (reducedfat) Coconut oil (virgin, organic) Fish oil (contaminate-free) Flax oil (not for cooking) Olive oil (extra virgin) Sesameseed oil *use all fats sparingly

	Dairy / Eggs	
	Low-fat dairy Eggs	

DIET PLAN 2 – DAILY FOODS

Meat / Fish		Vegetables	Fruits
Beef	Anchovies	Artichoke	Apple
Buffalo (Bison)	Clam Crab	Asparagus	Apricot
Elk	Crayfish	Avocado	Berries
Lamb	Herring	Bean sprouts	Cherries
Organ meats:	Lobster	Cauliflower	Coconut
Liver	Mussel	Carrot	Grapes
Kidney	Oyster	Celery	Nectarine
Heart	Perch	Collard greens	Peach
Pork(chops, ham)	Salmon	Corn	Pear
Wild game	Sardines	Green beans	Plum
Chicken (dark)	Scallop	Lettuce	
Leg and thigh	Shrimp	Olives	
Duck	Trout	Peas	
Goose	Tuna (dark)	Spinach	
Pheasant		Squash	
Turkey (dark)		Sweet potato	
Leg and thigh		Turnip	
		Turnip greens	

Grains	Beans*	Fats and oils
Whole grain breads	All	Butter (organic, full fat)
Whole grain cereals		Coconut oil (virgin)
Barley	*best if eaten with	
Cornmeal	flesh protein	Fish oil (contaminate-free)
Oat/Oatmeal	**Nuts and Seeds**	Flax oil (not for cooking)
Quinoa	All	
Rice:		Olive oil (extra virgin)
Basmati		Sesame seed oil
Brown	**Dairy / Eggs**	
Wild	Full-fat dairy	
Rye		
Wheat	Eggs (may not be a sufficient source of protein)	